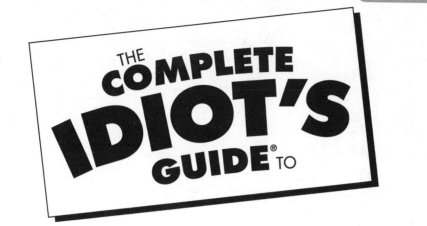

THE COMPLETE IDIOT'S GUIDE® TO

Fibromyalgia

Second Edition

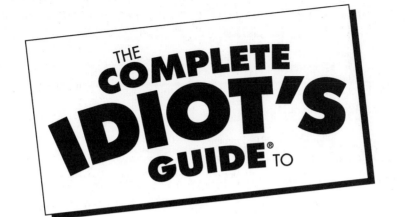

THE
COMPLETE
IDIOT'S
GUIDE® TO

Fibromyalgia

Second Edition

by Lynne Matallana
with Laurence A. Bradley, Ph.D.

ALPHA

A member of Penguin Group (USA) Inc.

This book is dedicated to the millions of people worldwide who are living with fibromyalgia. May there come a day when the pain of fibromyalgia is a distant memory, and until then may we support one another and encourage others to understand our challenges.

ALPHA BOOKS

Published by the Penguin Group

Penguin Group (USA) Inc., 375 Hudson Street, New York, New York 10014, USA

Penguin Group (Canada), 90 Eglinton Avenue East, Suite 700, Toronto, Ontario M4P 2Y3, Canada (a division of Pearson Penguin Canada Inc.)

Penguin Books Ltd., 80 Strand, London WC2R 0RL, England

Penguin Ireland, 25 St. Stephen's Green, Dublin 2, Ireland (a division of Penguin Books Ltd.)

Penguin Group (Australia), 250 Camberwell Road, Camberwell, Victoria 3124, Australia (a division of Pearson Australia Group Pty. Ltd.)

Penguin Books India Pvt. Ltd., 11 Community Centre, Panchsheel Park, New Delhi—110 017, India

Penguin Group (NZ), 67 Apollo Drive, Rosedale, North Shore, Auckland 1311, New Zealand (a division of Pearson New Zealand Ltd.)

Penguin Books (South Africa) (Pty.) Ltd., 24 Sturdee Avenue, Rosebank, Johannesburg 2196, South Africa

Penguin Books Ltd., Registered Offices: 80 Strand, London WC2R 0RL, England

Copyright © 2009 by Lynne Matallana

International Standard Book Number: 978-1-59257-833-7
Library of Congress Catalog Card Number: 2008931269

11   10   09   8   7   6   5   4   3   2   1

Interpretation of the printing code: The rightmost number of the first series of numbers is the year of the book's printing; the rightmost number of the second series of numbers is the number of the book's printing. For example, a printing code of 09-1 shows that the first printing occurred in 2009.

Printed in the United States of America

Note: This publication contains the opinions and ideas of its author. It is intended to provide helpful and informative material on the subject matter covered. It is sold with the understanding that the author and publisher are not engaged in rendering professional services in the book. If the reader requires personal assistance or advice, a competent professional should be consulted.

The author and publisher specifically disclaim any responsibility for any liability, loss, or risk, personal or otherwise, which is incurred as a consequence, directly or indirectly, of the use and application of any of the contents of this book.

Most Alpha books are available at special quantity discounts for bulk purchases for sales promotions, premiums, fund-raising, or educational use. Special books, or book excerpts, can also be created to fit specific needs.

For details, write: Special Markets, Alpha Books, 375 Hudson Street, New York, NY 10014.

Publisher: *Marie Butler-Knight*
Editorial Director/Acquiring Editor: *Mike Sanders*
Senior Managing Editor: *Billy Fields*
Development Editor: *Ginny Bess Munroe*
Senior Production Editor: *Janette Lynn*
Copy Editor: *Michael Dietsch*

Cartoonist: *Steve Barr*
Cover Designer: *Bill Thomas*
Book Designer: *Trina Wurst*
Indexer: *Heather McNeill*
Layout: *Brian Massey*
Proofreader: *John Etchison*

Contents at a Glance

Contents

Foreword

Fibromyalgia is a chronic disorder characterized by widespread pain and exquisite pain sensitivity that may produce high levels of suffering and greatly diminish your quality of life. These potentially negative effects are frequently compounded by inadequate knowledge of the physiologic abnormalities that contribute to the primary symptoms of the disorder. The inadequate knowledge also makes it difficult for many health-care professionals and patients to treat fibromyalgia as a chronic disorder. A large number of books have been published over the last 10 years regarding fibromyalgia, and a great deal of information is available on the Internet. Many of these sources provide helpful information about the current understanding of the pathophysiology of fibromyalgia as well as the medical and behavioral treatments that may produce symptom improvement. Until now, however, there have been no books devoted to educating patients about the ways they can actively self-manage their symptoms with the help of health-care professionals.

The Complete Idiot's Guide to Fibromyalgia, Second Edition, written by Ms. Lynne Matallana, president of the National Fibromyalgia Association, focuses primarily on helping persons with fibromyalgia understand and fully accept fibromyalgia. She wants readers to understand it is similar to other chronic illnesses, such as diabetes or rheumatoid arthritis, and is a disorder that cannot be cured by current medical or surgical treatments. Nevertheless, this book strongly emphasizes that, similar to patients with other chronic illnesses, individuals with fibromyalgia may learn to actively participate with their physicians and other health-care professionals, family members, and friends to manage their illness and produce optimal improvements in their quality of life. In other words, this book is an excellent guide for exchanging one's view of oneself as a passive recipient of treatments. The book will help you exchange views with a variety of people, including others who have little control of your symptoms, or an individual who is capable of developing a team of helpful persons who can identify self-management strategies that will best enhance your quality of life.

Readers of this book may be concerned that self-management is a term that really means "toughing it out" on one's own or suffering silently without support from others. This interpretation is entirely wrong. Instead, self-management is really a process of (a) identifying effective approaches to pharmacologic, behavioral (for example, exercise), and psychosocial treatment; and (b) identifying better methods of interacting with health professionals, family, and friends to improve physical and psychological health as well as your ability to perform productive and enjoyable activities of daily living. The latter process includes learning to alter deeply entrenched, negative patterns of behavior, thoughts, and emotional responses that contribute to a diminished quality of life. The approach advocated by Ms. Matallana is based on the premise that the best methods of self-management vary among individuals. Moreover, self-management of a chronic disorder, such as fibromyalgia, does not have a time limit. Instead, self-management is a process that goes on throughout your lifetime but may have to be changed over time to maintain the best possible quality of life.

This book presents helpful instructions and other tools that people with fibromyalgia can use to learn to self-manage their disorder. It also recognizes that self-management is difficult for most individuals. However, this book always maintains a very positive approach that includes great empathy for the problems that confront patients with fibromyalgia. It also contains detailed instructions on the behavioral and cognitive changes that highly motivated individuals may make to improve their health status and other dimensions of their lives.

—Laurence A. Bradley, Ph.D.

Introduction

Over the past decade the public, medical and scientific communities have come to better understand what it means to live with fibromyalgia. Although misperceptions still exist, fibromyalgia is now a subject that receives daily attention by the media, and continues to become of interest to educational institutions, professional organizations, businesses, and government agencies. Although fibromyalgia patients continue to have to search for knowledgeable health-care providers in their communities, and we haven't discovered the "magic bullet cure," having fibromyalgia is not as disheartening as it was in the past.

Even over the past few years there have been great strides made in the scientific understanding of this chronic pain disorder. As the science shows us that fibromyalgia is a condition of pain amplification in the nervous system, we are better able to discover new and improved treatments that will help patients to find a better quality of life. Whereas in the not so distant past people with fibromyalgia were living with what was considered an "invisible illness," today a new awareness exists and fibromyalgia is accepted as a life-altering disease that affects millions of people around the world.

I believe that the future continues to look brighter and people with fibromyalgia have more hope than ever before. However, we know that fibromyalgia remains a challenging disease and patients must continue to find ways to better self-manage their symptoms.

This book focuses on the importance of taking things a day at a time and working toward creating a lifestyle that will result in both emotional and physical well-being. Throughout this book you learn how to evaluate, develop, and implement techniques that will take you from being a patient who is desperate and miserable to becoming a happy, productive, healthier person—one who just happens to have fibromyalgia.

The journey of moving from being a fibromyalgia patient to a person who lives well despite fibromyalgia is not always easy. But throughout this book you will find information that will help you to discover ways to ensure that you will have a happier and healthier life. The information that is contained in this book will provide you with insights and techniques that will help you to become a fibromyalgia survivor!

How This Book Is Organized

To help you live better despite fibromyalgia, I've organized *The Complete Idiot's Guide to Fibromyalgia, Second Edition,* into a step-by-step process to help you develop a personalized self-management program. From diagnosis to ... a quality life beyond fibromyalgia.

Part 1: "Where Do I Start?"

Whether the onset of fibromyalgia was drawn out over a long period of time or as the result of a trauma (causing symptoms to virtually appear overnight), you will find yourself facing countless questions, wondering what methods will help you cope, and asking what will eventually improve the symptoms of this chronic pain condition. As you come to better understand this illness and accept the fact that although it is chronic in nature, you can take back control of your life, you will learn what options are available to help you. By developing your own self-management plan, you will be better able to manage your symptoms, discover what works best for you, and improve your outlook and overall quality of life.

In this part, you learn that life with fibromyalgia is like taking a journey into unknown territory. It can be frustrating and scary, but it can also give you the opportunity to learn and experience new things and make changes that will help improve both your emotional and physical health. You will be most successful if you take things a day at a time, focusing on setting realistic goals, approaching life with a positive attitude, and prioritizing and choosing to take the necessary steps to find improved overall health and well-being. There are ways to feel inspired by the journey you are about to take.

Part 2: "Who Can Help Me?"

The old adage "two heads are better than one" rings very true when it comes to fibromyalgia. Finding the right individuals to give you support and to provide the necessary medical expertise will ensure that you have an advantage when it comes to improving your health. Finding a balance between taking responsibility for your own health and also trusting in others who will become a part of your health-care team is vital. Learning when and how to ask for help will encourage others to want to be there when you need them and will allow you to rest assured that you have a team that is working together assisting you to get better.

You must remember that your illness affects everyone around you. It is important that you are sensitive to their needs, too. By working together you will be able to find ways to modify and improve the many aspects of your family's life that may have changed. Good communication and the willingness to compromise will help everyone adjust and eventually feel comfortable with these new challenges.

Part 3: "What Are the Treatment Options?"

Although there isn't a cure for fibromyalgia or even a tried-and-true treatment protocol that works for everyone, there is a series of pharmacological and complementary alternatives that have been shown to help reduce many of the symptoms of fibromyalgia and its overlapping conditions. Just like many things in life, finding the answers to your questions may take time and patience, but the important thing is to recognize that you do have options. By evaluating them, deciding where your comfort level is, and then preceding with them in a step-by-step manner, you will have positive results. It's important to always remind yourself that others have pursued this journey before you and have found that the path leads to helpful answers and new hope for an improved future.

To learn what options you have and how to make educated decisions, this part gives you an extensive outline of the many treatment options that make up a multidisciplinary approach for treating fibromyalgia. From drugs that help alleviate symptoms to lifestyle changes that can reduce stress and change the way you approach life, the options are many and the choices are yours.

Part 4: "What Can I Do to Feel Better?"

As you begin to learn about treatment options, you'll learn that you have to let go of negativity and learn how to balance your life with lifestyle changes, such as a good night's sleep and diet and exercise that are customized for you. You also learn that you must deal with stress and anxiety. This part teaches you how to stop trying to be perfect and how to find help when you need it. It also provides 25 tips that make you feel better, help you rid your life of negativity and stress, and teach you how to achieve a more balanced life.

Part 5: "What Will the Future Be Like?"

There are times when life with fibromyalgia will seem overwhelming and uncertain. The fact that this illness can wax and wane might make you wonder if the future will continue to challenge you with cycles of symptoms. Improvements may not come as quickly as you would like, and it may test your ability to stay strong and hopeful. Despite your temptation to feel despondent, you can rest assured that the medical community is moving forward in their understanding of the causes of fibromyalgia and will soon have new and improved treatments. Research is expanding and more and more people are becoming interested in finding the answers to questions that will provide patients with new options. Specific medications are close to being approved to treat fibromyalgia, and a new momentum to find additional pharmacological treatments has begun. We are living in a time that has more hope than ever before. It is important to surround yourself with people who are optimistic and know that new ideas and new treatments will become a part of your future.

This book also includes a glossary and two additional appendixes containing resource information and a forms section, which allows you to keep contact information, organize your medical records, create checklists, and record personal thoughts and information.

Bonus Information

In addition to the main text of *The Complete Idiot's Guide to Fibromyalgia, Second Edition*, you'll find other types of useful information. Here's how to recognize these features:

> ### Healthy Alternative
> These suggestions will identify options to help you in your quest for better health.

> ### def•i•ni•tion
> Here's where you will find the definitions that help explain those hard-to-understand medical terms.

> ### Fast Fact
> These are factual tidbits that will help you better understand pertinent information.

> ### Pain Signal
> These notes are designed to help you recognize things that might be harmful to you and your health.

> ### Picture This/Lessons Learned
> These personal stories have been shared to help you better understand certain situations and to help motivate you in your pursuit to overcome fibromyalgia.

Acknowledgments

When one door closes, another one opens.

Life as I knew it came to a screeching halt in 1995. As my body became consumed with the pain and exhaustion of fibromyalgia, all I could imagine was a future of misery and frustration. Never could I have guessed that from this suffering I would find a whole new way of looking at life. Never did I imagine that this experience would allow me to meet some of the most remarkable people I have ever known and that they would teach me the power of compassion and fortitude. The writing of this book was inspired by all who live well despite their pain, those who pursue the scientific truths to better understand this illness, and those who provide us with support, care, and unconditional love.

This book would not have been possible without the help of the following people: my husband, Richard, who has always believed in me and provided me with love and support so that I could follow my dreams; my mom, Joanne, who during my school years motivated, helped, and encouraged me as I suffered over every word I would write, preparing me for all the writing I would do in the future; and my brother, Craig, who has so much creative talent that he can take a concept and turn it into an informational picture or an inspirational piece of art.

Stephan Severance, M.D., and Norman Simon, M.D., who believed in me and understood that fibromyalgia is real. Each was willing to dedicate his concern, time, and medical talents to find the path that would help improve my health. Members of my "daily caregiver team," who became dear friends, Ila and Eve, both of whom spent hours encouraging me and helping me to understand. And to my longtime friends who are true friends, Leslie, June, Leisa, and Dagmar.

To the people who are now the body and soul of the National Fibromyalgia Association. My cofounder, Karen Lee Richards, who has put her concern for others with fibromyalgia as a lifelong priority. Errol Landy, who has dedicated his time and energies to becoming invaluable to the FM community and is like a brother to me. Karin Amour, Nancy Derby, and Sharon Squires, who have given completely of themselves to ensure that the fibromyalgia community will have an organization that supports and fights for the needs of people with fibromyalgia everywhere.

The experts who continue to find time in their incredibly busy lives to support the fibromyalgia community and who enthusiastically gave of themselves to help me with this book:

Robert Bennett, M.D.

Daniel Clauw, M.D.

Peter Farvolden, Ph.D.

Mark Pellegrino, M.D.

I. Jon Russell, M.D.

Dennis Turk, Ph.D.

Daniel Wallace, M.D.

David Williams, Ph.D.

The staff and volunteers at the National Fibromyalgia Association, who had to "hold down the fort" while I took time to write this book. And to those who continue to give more than they take in life: Syvilla Fry; Vicki and Alonzo Pedrin; Dory Ford; Carlos Valcercel; Barbara Ebberts; Jessie Jones, Ph.D.; and John and Linda Benner.

To Scott E. Davis, Esq., and Joshua Potter, Esq., who were instrumental in helping me compile the information on disability.

And special thanks, gratitude, and admiration go to the book's medical editors, who gave of their time, expertise, compassion, and brilliance to ensure that this book would provide unique information and ameliorate the lives of people with fibromyalgia. I was honored to work with each of you.

Laurence A. Bradley, Ph.D. ... *who trusted me*

Stuart Silverman, M.D., FACP, FACR ... *who taught me*

Muhammad B. Yunus, M.D., FACP, FACR, FRCPE ... *who supported me*

Trademarks

All terms mentioned in this book that are known to be or are suspected of being trademarks or service marks have been appropriately capitalized. Alpha Books and Penguin Group (USA) Inc. cannot attest to the accuracy of this information. Use of a term in this book should not be regarded as affecting the validity of any trademark or service mark.

Part 1

Where Do I Start?

Whether the onset of your fibromyalgia was drawn out over a long period of time or as the result of a trauma—causing symptoms to virtually appear overnight—you will find yourself facing countless questions, wondering what methods will help you cope and eventually help improve your symptoms of this chronic pain condition. By developing a self-management plan, you will better manage your symptoms, discover what works best for you, and improve your outlook and overall quality of life.

In this part, you will learn that life with fibromyalgia is like taking a journey into unknown territory. It can be frustrating and scary, but it can also give you the opportunity to learn and experience new things and make changes that will help improve both your emotional and physical health. You will be most successful if you take things a day at a time, focusing on setting realistic goals, approaching life with a positive attitude, and prioritizing and choosing the necessary steps to find improved overall health and well-being.

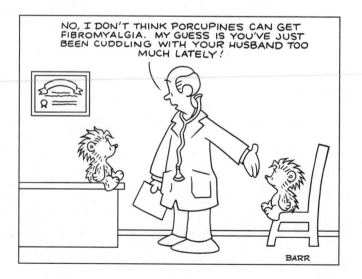

Could It Be Fibromyalgia?

In This Chapter

- ◆ Living with fibromyalgia
- ◆ Knowing who can get fibromyalgia
- ◆ Learning the symptoms of fibromyalgia
- ◆ Finding out if you have fibromyalgia

It wasn't long ago that only a handful of researchers were familiar with the term *fibromyalgia*. Throughout much of the last century, people complaining of chronic pain throughout their body were often diagnosed with "fibrositis," a condition thought to be an inflammatory disease of the muscles. But in the 1970s, a small group of researchers rejected the idea that this kind of pain was of an inflammatory nature and began writing about the association of chronic muscle pain, tender points, and sleep abnormalities. A new understanding was developing for this group of specific symptoms, and the term *fibrositis* was no longer appropriate. In 1976, this group of symptoms was given a new name: *fibromyalgia*—a word that defined the symptoms of and gave credibility to a large group of people who had been struggling to learn what was causing them to feel the way they did. This new name helped unite a group of individuals who at one time felt isolated and alone.

At last the foundation for a better understanding of fibromyalgia had been estab-lished. Today, our knowledge of fibromyalgia is growing fast and the number of researchers involved in solving the mysteries of this condition continues to increase. Although we still have much to learn about fibromyalgia, awareness and compre-hension are rapidly increasing, and the answers to many of our questions about this chronic pain disorder are in our future.

Experiencing Fibromyalgia

I remember the exact moment when I knew there was something very wrong with me. It was like a tornado whirling around me, making me feel terrified and completely disoriented. Pain surged throughout my entire body. It was like the tornado had picked me up and then slammed me to the ground. The reality was that I was lying face down on my bathroom floor, unaware of how I had gotten there, desperately trying to bring things back into focus. But all I could concentrate on was the sensa-tion that my entire body was on fire and my insides were tied in knots. The cold tiles of the bathroom floor coaxed me back to consciousness, and as I tried to stand up, I realized that my husband was with me, frantic with concern.

That morning I had had a routine laparoscopy for endometriosis. I was so excited about having the procedure because I was looking forward to answers that would help free my future of the horrendous monthly episodes of headaches, cramping, and excruciating pain. But only a few hours after the procedure, I felt worse than I could have ever imagined. Now the pain was everywhere: sharp and cramping, but aching and burning. It made me want to cry out in misery.

My husband got me back into bed and I tried to explain to him what I was feeling. Throughout my life I had always been "sensitive" to pain, but I had refused to let it slow me down. I had come to the conclusion that everyone probably felt like that, and it was just something that I, like everyone else, had to put up with. But now some-thing told me that I did feel pain more than others. The doctor had told me that I might experience some discomfort following the procedure, but this was intolerable pain. As always I started to feel guilty, trying to understand why I was such a wimp and couldn't tolerate pain like others. But my guilt slipped away as I begged my hus-band to help me understand what was happening to me.

Over the next few weeks I began experiencing an array of symptoms. Each one made the situation more distressing, but my doctor told me that I was fine, and that the symptoms would go away in time. Two months later, sitting in a fog at our company's annual Christmas party, I was still wondering, "When am I going to feel better?" Little did I know that this was just the beginning. Over the next two years I was going to have to fight to find the answers and dig deep within myself to find the strength and courage to deal with whatever each day brought me. It was a time in my life that I would never want to revisit, but it was also a time when I learned a lot about myself—and discovered a new purpose for my life.

Fibromyalgia Is Pain

Fibromyalgia is real. For those who have experienced chronic widespread pain and nagging fatigue, along with the spectrum of other "fibro" symptoms, there is no debate over its existence. The pain is not something that we imagine, nor is it something we can "will away." Fibromyalgia is a condition that involves chronic pain amplification that is caused by *neuroendocrine abnormalities*.

When living with fibromyalgia, trying to convince others that your pain is real can be as frustrating as the pain itself! When friends and family look at you and say, "… But you don't look sick!" their lack of understanding and support can be daunting. So the everyday challenges of living with fibromyalgia go beyond the actual symptoms. Learning to live with an "invisible" illness not only means searching for treatment options and developing a lifestyle that helps decrease symptoms, it also means remaining positive and educating those who are skeptical about your diagnosis.

def•i•ni•tion

Neuroendocrine abnormalities refer to neurological and hormonal/chemical irregularities that cause disordered sensory processing, resulting in pain and other symptoms.

Fortunately, the medical community has begun to identify and better understand fibromyalgia's causes and treatments. Although the constellation of symptoms, now known as fibromyalgia syndrome, has been referenced throughout history (going back as far as biblical times), it is considered a relatively new diagnosis. It is only within the past 20 to 30 years that research has advanced our understanding of the condition. Although there are currently no laboratory tests, x-rays, or definitive markers to test for fibromyalgia, more and more research is identifying physical abnormalities in people with fibromyalgia. It will take time for it to be accepted and understood by the public, and for the medical community to advance its research to separate theory from fact.

Fast Fact _____

Great historical figures, such as Red Cross founder Florence Nightingale (1820–1910) and scientist Alfred Bernhard Nobel (1833–1896), probably had fibromyalgia. Nobel wrote, "Sometimes I cannot sleep a moment for an entire week and thus have developed an indescribable nerve irritation."

It's Not All in Your Head!

For those of us diagnosed with fibromyalgia, the future is not bleak. Fibromyalgia should not define your existence or mean that quality of life is not possible. Although living with this chronic illness can be challenging, it is important to focus on the positive and to keep in mind that treatment options exist. The future holds much promise for a better understanding of this previously misunderstood condition and, even though there are still naysayers who believe that fibromyalgia is "all in your head," the vast majority of the medical community has abandoned that myth and has instead begun to focus on determining which therapies are effective for patients. Although there are still people who have never heard of fibromyalgia, the Food and Drug Administration estimates that it affects between 8 and 10 million people in the United States.

Chronic pain can have far-reaching consequences upon individuals, families, and society as a whole. There is now national recognition that scientific understanding of the process of pain is needed. For people with fibromyalgia, this means that there is hope for a better future.

def•i•ni•tion _____

A **multidisciplinary approach** is when a patient selects and utilizes the expertise of different specialists who practice both traditional and nontraditional medical approaches to treat the patient's symptoms.

In the meantime, concentrate on the current treatment options that make up a _multidisciplinary approach_ to living with fibromyalgia. When you become educated about this approach and learn how to adapt to a healthier lifestyle, you will be taking the steps necessary to recapture the happy, productive existence you enjoyed before you began experiencing symptoms. This book focuses on how you can become an active self-manager of your fibromyalgia and have a better quality of life!

Fibro-My-What?

The name *fibromyalgia* comes from the Latin words *fibro* (fibrous tissues), *my* (muscles), and *algia* (pain). Together, these words describe the main symptom of fibromyalgia: painful muscles, tendons, and ligaments. However, widespread pain throughout the soft tissues of the body is only one of the symptoms considered part of the syndrome. Chronic pain is also accompanied by fatigue, disordered sleep, stiffness, numbness, cognitive difficulties, anxiety, muscle weakness, and sensitivity to light and sound.

Originally, fibromyalgia was known as *fibrositis*, a term first used in a 1904 lecture by Sir William Gowers. The disease's name was changed to fibromyalgia in 1976; in 1990 the American College of Rheumatology established the existing criteria for diagnosis. Gowers and his colleagues believed that fibrositis was caused by inflammation of the fibrous tissues of the body. However, the research of the 1970s and 1980s proved that there was no inflammation of the muscles. The new research focus has become central nervous system dysfunction.

Fast Fact

Although fibromyalgia is often considered an arthritis-related condition, research has shown that it is not a form of arthritis, but is actually a neuroendocrine illness. Abnormal levels of hormones and chemicals involved in pain processing in the central nervous system are thought to result in pain amplification.

People with fibromyalgia have physical abnormalities that result in pain amplification, causing pain to be perceived even when they are exposed to sensations that would not normally be painful. For example, you might find that certain clothing, a soft touch on your arm, or even a bright light can cause extreme pain and fatigue. By developing a lifestyle that reduces stress and includes structured sleep habits and avoidance of activities that increase pain, it is possible to reduce the amount of discomfort you experience.

Although there currently is no cure for fibromyalgia, the symptoms can be managed. By learning what it is and how to develop your own self-management program, you can reduce its effect on your life and become a fibromyalgia survivor!

The Pain Is in the Brain

Over the past 20 years, research has shown that people with fibromyalgia are sick in the head. That doesn't mean they've imagined their pain and fatigue! It means there are many physiological abnormalities taking place in the brain. For example, we now know that people with fibromyalgia have decreased blood flow to certain areas of the brain that help modulate pain signals sent from the spinal cord. Researchers have also found genetic markers that may signal the illness and, most recently, mutation in the regulatory region of the serotonin transporter gene.

One of the most important research findings has been duplicated in multiple studies. This research shows that people with fibromyalgia have three to four times the normal level of substance P, a neurotransmitter in the central nervous system that is involved in pain processing. And more recently, researchers have found deficiencies in growth hormone as well as low levels of insulin-like growth factor-1 (IGF), which is also called somatomedin C, a hormone that promotes bone and muscle growth.

Other major findings show that people with fibromyalgia have low levels of important neurochemicals, or organic substances located in the brain that are involved in neurological processes. These include ...

◆ Serotonin, a nervous system chemical messenger (neurotransmitter). Serotonin plays important roles in feelings of well-being, modulating pain, and promoting deep sleep.

◆ Norepinephrine, dopamine, and cortisol, which are important stress hormones.

◆ The muscle-cell chemicals phosphocreatine and adenosine triphosphate (ATP). These chemicals regulate calcium in muscle cells, which helps them contract and relax.

As research continues to grow, it will be impossible for anyone to doubt the physical abnormalities that occur within the brain and body of a person with fibromyalgia!

Who It Affects

Fibromyalgia is often referred to as a "woman's illness" because 75 to 85 percent of the people who receive a diagnosis are women. The truth is, however, it does affect millions of people, and anyone (including men and children) can get it. Fibromyalgia does not discriminate based on sex, age, race, or nationality. It is estimated that 3–6 percent of the world's population has fibromyalgia and that millions of people remain undiagnosed.

Fast Fact _____

More people in the United States have fibromyalgia than lupus (1.5 million people), multiple sclerosis (400,000 people), and Parkinson's disease (500,000 people) combined.

We know that most people develop fibromyalgia symptoms in their 30s or 40s, but it is not uncommon to be diagnosed in the 20s or 50s … or at any other age. Elementary school–aged children have been diagnosed with fibromyalgia, though for decades researchers did not suspect children could develop the disorder. It is not uncommon, however, for adults diagnosed with fibromyalgia to remember having unexplained symptoms for many years—even reaching back into their childhood. In the United States, one out of every 50 Americans has fibromyalgia. It exists in industrialized countries, third-world countries, and even isolated populations such as the Amish.

Although not as many men are diagnosed with fibromyalgia as women, this does not mean that men do not suffer the same intense symptoms. Many explanations have been given for the gender disparity (such as variations in hormones and pain sensitivity) but to date, there is no definitive reason. We do know that men and women differ biologically and that women have hormonally dependent pain traits. The important thing is to be aware that men do develop the syndrome and that they, too, can benefit from learning a multidisciplinary approach.

Fast Fact _____

Women tend to be better at translating nonverbal signals of communication then men. This may make them better able to recognize and express their pain. Women are usually more willing to acknowledge and talk about their physical discomforts than men.

The Symptoms

Fibromyalgia is classified as a syndrome because it is a collection of symptoms and overlapping conditions. Because it can mimic other illnesses and coexist with other diseases such as lupus, rheumatoid arthritis, and even cancer, fibromyalgia is difficult to diagnose. As the original research collaborators found, there is a group of complaints that are consistent with the majority of people with fibromyalgia. Although each person does not necessarily have all the symptoms, individuals often experience many of the symptoms at one time or another.

In the following chart, place a check mark next to each symptom you have experienced. When you see a health-care professional, take a copy of this list to share the information with him or her.

Symptoms and Overlapping Conditions

Overlapping Condition	Had in Past	Have Now	Date of Onset
Body-wide Muscle and Joint Pain			
Fatigue			
Altered Sleep			
Stiffness			
Dizziness (Balance Problems)			
Sensitivity to Environmental Factors (light, sound, smells, temperature)			
Temporomandibular Joint (TMJ) Dysfunction			
Chronic Fatigue Syndrome			
Headaches			
Migraines			
Anxiety/Panic Attacks			
Irritable Bowel Syndrome			
Paresthesia (numbness and tingling)			
Allergies and Chemical Sensitivities			
Restless Leg Syndrome			
Dry Mouth and Eyes			
Skin Rashes and Irritations			
Cognitive Impairments			
Vulvodynia			
Endometriosis			
Interstitial Cystitis			

Overlapping Condition	Had in Past	Have Now	Date of Onset
Painful Menstrual Periods			
Mitral Valve Prolapse			
Neurally Mediated Hypotension			
Ringing in Ears			
Depression			
Myofascial Regional Pain Syndrome			
Raynaud's Phenomenon			
Irritable Bladder			
Reflex Sympathetic Dystrophy Syndrome			
Hypermobility			
Hypoglycemia			
Hypothyroid			
Carpal Tunnel Syndrome			

The main symptom or chief complaint is constant widespread pain, above and below the waist and on both sides of the body. Individuals with fibromyalgia often feel like they have the flu and are completely out of energy! The pain can be described as stabbing, burning, tingling, aching, or even cramping. People with fibromyalgia may experience sleepless nights and awaken feeling even more tired than they did when they went to bed. Many people with fibromyalgia experience super sensitivity to touch, light, sound, and even the weather. Cognitive difficulties are quite common and are often referred to as *fibro fog.*

def•i•ni•tion

Many people with fibromyalgia experience cognitive difficulties, making it tricky for them to verbally express their thoughts. Oftentimes in the middle of a conversation, **fibro fog** causes them to lose their train of thought. The term fibro fog is used by people with fibromyalgia because this symptom makes them feel like their thinking is foggy.

Because fibromyalgia will cause you to experience multiple symptoms that ebb and flow, and may even seem to appear and disappear at random, at times it becomes difficult to lead a routine life. When symptoms appear, they can disrupt your plans, expectations, and even your lifestyle. The intensity of one's symptoms can also vary from mild to extreme. It is frustrating to feel less pain one day and more the next—especially when you cannot understand the reason behind the increase.

Sometimes you can figure out what causes the pain to "flare up," but at other times, it is best to spend less energy trying to analyze what made the symptoms worse, and instead to concentrate on what can be done to make your body *hardier* overall. It is important to get an early diagnosis and begin to identify your symptoms and decide what treatment options you want to try.

def•i•ni•tion

When your health-care professional uses the term **hardier,** he or she means that you should work toward becoming healthier, stronger, and more capable of surviving unfavorable situations. The result is a reduction of symptoms and an overall improvement in your physical and emotional condition.

Fibromyalgia Symptom Frequency

It is not unusual for a person with fibromyalgia to experience multiple symptoms and a variety of other chronic conditions. An explanation for this is that these syndromes share a common pathophysiological mechanism. In other words, unlike illnesses that have structural damage (such as cancer or a broken leg) or a psychiatric component (such as schizophrenia), these illnesses have neurological and endocrine system abnormalities that cause hypersensitivity and dysfunction within the central nervous system. Because this is a whole new way of looking at and understanding certain illnesses, researchers must accept a new direction for research.

Many of the symptoms of fibromyalgia occur in people who do not have the disorder. It is important to find out what your symptoms mean. The following list describes the frequency at which some of the symptoms and overlapping conditions affect people with fibromyalgia. Additional research will be necessary in order for us to understand to what degree patients experience all the symptoms and overlapping conditions.

Fibromyalgia Symptom Frequency

Symptom	Frequency (%)
❏ Widespread muscle and joint pain	100%
❏ Fatigue	80%
❏ Sleep difficulties	75%
❏ Numbness and tingling	64%
❏ Dizziness	60%
❏ Swollen feeling in tissues	40%
Aggravating Factors of Pain	
❏ Cold temperature	80%
❏ Anxiety	80%
❏ Poor sleep	76%
❏ Stress	63%
❏ Overuse or trauma	62%
❏ Physical inactivity	48%
❏ Noise	24%
Overlapping Conditions/Symptoms	
❏ Chronic fatigue syndrome	64%
❏ Irritable bowel syndrome	60%
❏ Multiple chemical sensitivity	55%
❏ Headaches	53%
❏ Dizziness	47%
❏ Primary dysmenorrhea	45%
❏ Restless legs syndrome	31%
❏ Female urethral syndrome	12%
❏ Dry mouth	12%
❏ Temporomandibular dysfunction	Common*
❏ Periodic limb movement disorder	Common*
❏ Cognitive impairment	Common

These conditions are common in clinical practice, but there is no specific data regarding their frequency. Adapted from Muhammad B. Yunus, M.D.'s chapter in Textbook of Fibromyalgia and Other Non-Neuropathic Pain Syndromes.

Dr. Muhammad Yunus has identified a group of chronic conditions that have similar features and often overlap in a single individual. The following diagram shows members of what he calls Central Sensitivity Syndromes (CSS).

Central Sensitivity Syndromes (CSS) share overlapping features and a common biophysiological mechanism of neuroendocrine dysfunction/central sensitivity. (Adapted from Muhammad B. Yunus, M.D., Professor of Medicine at the College of Medicine at Peoria, with permission.)

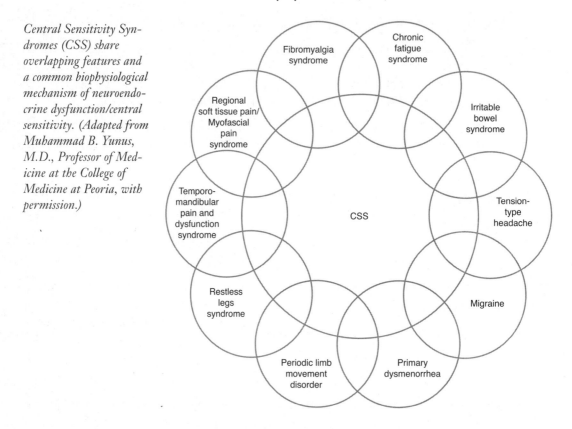

How Fibromyalgia Is Diagnosed

The diagnostic criteria for fibromyalgia were established in 1990 by the American College of Rheumatology (ACR). The ACR explained that fibromyalgia is "… a painful, but not articular [not present in the joints], condition predominantly involving muscles and is the most common cause of chronic widespread musculoskeletal pain." In 1993, the World Health Organization held the Second World Congress on Myofascial Pain and Fibromyalgia, and officially recognized the ACR's criteria for diagnosis in the Copenhagen Declaration.

The ACR's criteria of classification of fibromyalgia were based on a blinded, multi-center study that evaluated 11 symptom variables, including sleep disturbances, frequent headaches, and stress levels.

The study reported two decisive findings, which are now the basis of diagnosis:

◆ Widespread pain was present in 98 percent of fibromyalgia patients, compared with 69 percent of the control group. *Widespread pain* is defined as pain in the left and right sides of the body and above and below the waist, as well as axial skeletal pain (such as in the neck, front or back chest, and lower back).

◆ Pain in 11 of 18 *tender points* was reported on digital palpation ("tender" is not the same as painful); 88.4 percent of fibromyalgia patients had widespread pain in combination with pain in 11 of 18 tender points as described.

def•i•ni•tion

Tender points are areas of muscle or other soft tissues that are extremely sensitive to pressure stimulation. Most healthy individuals experience pain in only a small number of tender points. However, people diagnosed with fibromyalgia experience pain in 11 or more tender points.

Therefore, if you have a history of widespread pain for more than three months and the health-care professional finds pain in 11 or more tender points upon physical examination, a diagnosis of fibromyalgia can be made.

Although these criteria for diagnosis lack a specific "marker" for laboratory testing (such as a blood test, urine test, x-ray, and so on) and have been described as subjective, most researchers agree that they have been a beneficial tool for clinical research. They also point out that many other illnesses do not have definitive laboratory tests to prove their diagnoses. For now, tender points have been found to be very consistent sites for diagnosing individuals with fibromyalgia. As we better understand the cause(s) of fibromyalgia, new diagnostic criteria may emerge.

During a diagnosis, the health-care professional will press firmly on 18 (a total of nine pairs of) designated tender points located in the following areas:

◆ The left or right side of the back of the neck, directly below the hairline

◆ The left or right side of the front of the neck, above the collarbone (clavicle)

◆ The left or right side of the chest, right below the collarbone

- The left or right side of the upper back, near where the neck and shoulder join

- The left or right side of the spine in the upper back between the shoulder blades (scapulae)

- The inside of either arm, where it bends at the elbow

- The left or right side of the lower back, right below the waist

- Either side of the buttocks right under the hipbones

- On the fat pad over the kneecaps

Tender points diagram for diagnosis.

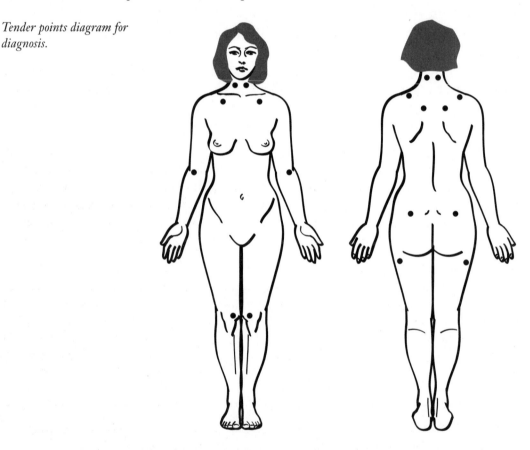

If 11 or more tender points are reported to be painful, the health-care professional may make a fibromyalgia diagnosis. Although these tender points are helpful in the diagnosis of fibromyalgia, they do not determine the severity of fibromyalgia symptoms.

Causes of Fibromyalgia

Many of our medical questions are answered after technology develops that allows us to see things more clearly. With today's new functional imaging techniques, researchers are actually able to take pictures of a functioning brain. In studies that have compared the brain of a person with fibromyalgia to a brain of someone who does not have fibromyalgia, researchers found that sensory input was altered or even malfunctioning in the fibromyalgia patient's brain. In other words, a fibromyalgic brain works differently than a healthy person's brain; the result is a miscommunication of pain signals.

This type of study has also shown that people with fibromyalgia have decreased levels of blood flow to the region of the brain that processes pain. But why do fibromyalgia patients have disordered sensory processing? The medical community suspects that there is a genetic predisposition to the illness. It appears that fibromyalgia runs in families, being more common among siblings and children of people who have fibromyalgia.

Many people report that their symptoms developed after a triggering event such as an accident or injury, viral infection, surgery, emotional or physical stress, or even exposure to certain drugs or chemicals. Fibromyalgia that has a quick onset after a car accident or physical injury is referred to as *post-traumatic fibromyalgia*. A large portion of the medical community accepts the current evidence that shows 35 to 65 percent of people develop fibromyalgia symptoms after experiencing a physical trauma.

Fast Fact

In a study published in 1997, Dan Buskila, M.D., of Israel, followed 161 people with traumatic injuries. Of those 161 people, 102 had neck injuries (whiplash), and 59 had leg fractures. The final evaluations showed that the people who had neck injuries developed fibromyalgia 22 percent of the time, whereas people with the leg injuries developed fibromyalgia only 2 percent of the time. This study is often referenced to prove that fibromyalgia can be triggered by traumatic injuries.

Research has shown that a very high number of people are diagnosed with fibromyalgia after car accidents and other injuries (see Chapter 11). Some believe that the accident (or other trauma) may cause a disturbance in how the central nervous system works, resulting in pain amplification. It is thought that the abnormalities in the central nervous system include imbalances or alterations in certain chemicals and hormones, which lead to increased pain perception. Although physical trauma seems to be the most commonly noted reason for symptom onset, emotional stress can also be a trigger. Others cannot identify a specific cause for the onset of symptoms and note that symptoms developed gradually over time.

Another area that has received a lot of attention as a possible cause of fibromyalgia is disordered sleep. People with fibromyalgia often have trouble getting to sleep, staying asleep, or getting into the deep levels of sleep that are needed to feel refreshed in the morning. Although there is no debate over the fact that people with fibromyalgia experience sleep difficulties, whether this is a cause of fibromyalgia or is just another symptom of the illness is still being evaluated.

Because fibromyalgia affects people in different ways, there have been many different ideas about its cause(s). Other explanations have included nutritional deficiencies, immune system dysfunction, psychiatric causes, yeast infections, environmental toxins, chronic infections, changes in muscle metabolism, lack of exercise, thyroid conditions, and Chiari malformation. Some have even claimed that fibromyalgia does not exist. Most researchers, however, believe that fibromyalgia is a medical entity and that it probably has multiple causes.

Taking Control and Changing Your Perception

To improve your life with fibromyalgia, you need to find a level of control that allows you to improve your symptoms, your attitude, and your total quality of life. The control that you find, however, is not the kind of control that gives you complete power over a situation—but the kind that allows you to feel comfortable and happy in a situation. For example, right now you might feel that you have lost the ability to participate in an athletic activity that you once enjoyed. With time, however, you can come to the point where you feel that you have control over the situation. Instead of dwelling on the fact that you cannot play tennis twice a week, you can remind yourself that now you enjoy swimming twice a week.

A change in perception is crucial to the quality of your future. Finding balance is actually a way of finding control. In later chapters, I discuss the importance of a balanced life and how to develop traits that help you control your situation—even if

> **Healthy Alternative**
>
> When I was first diagnosed with fibromyalgia, I felt that my entire life was out of control. By picking only one issue to deal with per day—or even, at first, per week—I didn't feel as overwhelmed as I did when I was trying to "fix" many aspects of my health at one time.

some of them appear to sound contradictory. For example, if you practice *perseverance*, doing so does not mean that you cannot also practice *patience*. You can ask for help, and this does not make you weak. You may even find that less can be more—doing one task well can be more rewarding than undertaking five tasks that you do not do so well!

Picture This/Lessons Learned

Picture This:

My doctor said my blood test showed that I was dehydrated and that I needed to greatly increase the amount of water I drank in a day. I started keeping a bottle of water with me at all times. Of course this isn't that difficult to do, but I was resentful that I had to always pay attention to where my water bottle was and whether I had drunk enough of the bland stuff. To top it off, I honestly didn't believe that it was going to make a difference in how I felt. I felt the situation was out of my control, which made me unhappy.

After I realized that the additional water did make me feel better—fewer headaches, fewer bowel problems, less dry skin, and so on—I was much more willing to make the extra effort. I did my own taste test and found a great-tasting water. Sometimes I even put the water in a crystal wine glass to make myself feel special, even though I was just drinking water! I found ways to feel more in control of the situation and not only did the results make me feel less frustrated, I also benefited by becoming *hardier*.

Lessons Learned:

Here are some simple ways to make improvements for a hardier life:

- Be willing to try simple alternatives. Even small changes can make a difference.
- If you have to do something to improve your health, find ways to make the improvements more enjoyable for you.
- Pay attention to small symptoms, such as digestive tract problems, rashes, headaches, bruising, and shortness of breath, that may be part of your fibromyalgia or an expression of a bigger problem.

What to Do Next

This chapter presented a lot of information. Armed with information, your journey through diagnosis, acceptance, and treatment will be much easier. The following chapters will guide and assist you in creating a self-management plan to help you better understand your chronic illness and develop a symptom management program that will ensure an improved quality of life. Remember: you are not alone!

Millions of other people are dealing with fibromyalgia on a daily basis—and there are many others who are deeply concerned about people with fibromyalgia. They are creating support systems, dedicating their lives to fibromyalgia research, and developing new treatments that will bring relief to those who currently suffer. Never before has there been so much interest in helping people with fibromyalgia. Never before has there been so much hope.

The Least You Need to Know

- Fibromyalgia is a real medical entity that causes multiple symptoms, including widespread body pain, fatigue, and sleep disturbances in an estimated 8 to 10 million people in the United States.

- Fibromyalgia affects men, women, and children of all ages, ethnicities, and economic levels.

- Currently we do not know if there is a definitive cause for fibromyalgia, nor is there a cure—but there are many ways those with the syndrome can improve their quality of life.

- We know more about the causes of and treatment options for fibromyalgia than ever before—and there is much hope for helping people with fibromyalgia in the future.

2

Fibromyalgia and Acceptance

In This Chapter

- ◆ Learning to accept fibromyalgia to reduce symptoms
- ◆ Finding balance in your life
- ◆ Discovering the 10 goals of acceptance
- ◆ Defining the stages of acceptance

Whether you have had fibromyalgia for a long time or have just recently been diagnosed, you can become a fibromyalgia survivor! When you can think about your illness and realize that you have learned from the experience and that you are a better person because of living with fibromyalgia, you will then know that you have not only accepted the illness, but you have become a survivor.

This chapter discusses how you can accept the disease without giving in to it. After you accept the disease, you need to learn how you can find balance and develop survival skills. This chapter teaches you how.

Developing Survival Skills

One of the most important things you need to learn after your fibromyalgia diagnosis is that you can manage this illness. Motivated individuals, working with concerned and knowledgeable health-care professionals, can experience significant improvements in their symptoms and quality of life. If, however, you expect it to be an all-or-nothing situation, you will not get results. If you look for a health-care professional who has a magic wand or a manufacturer that has the magic potion, your search will be lengthy—and frustrating. By accepting your illness and learning ways to improve your quality of life, however, you may discover that some extraordinarily positive things can come out of this incredibly difficult experience.

Healthy Alternative

The term "acceptance" does not mean that you just roll over and give up. Instead, if you accept the fact that you do have a chronic pain illness and you commit yourself to making an effort—whatever you can do at that particular moment to improve your situation—you will take back control of your life and become a fibromyalgia survivor.

No Pain, No Gain

Living with a chronic illness like fibromyalgia can help you learn some of life's most important lessons. It really is true that adversity can strengthen you and help you become a better human being. You might lose certain abilities, and you might even feel like you are not the same person, but with the right approach and attitude you can gain more than you lose.

Patients often comment that fibromyalgia teaches them how to better prioritize their lives. People are often preoccupied with many things that aren't really important, but fibromyalgia patients need to reserve their energy for the things that really count. This new lifestyle can be a way to simplify, reduce stress, and increase focus.

Shirley Boone, wife of singer Pat Boone, once told me that fibromyalgia gave her the ability to be a better caregiver when her grandson sustained life-threatening injuries after falling three stories through a skylight at his condominium. She believes that her own health trials helped her to connect with Ryan, spending weeks sitting next to bed while he lay in a coma. She felt an overwhelming need to be with him and support him while he slowly, miraculously started to heal and regain his life.

Picture This/Lessons Learned

Picture This:

When I first became ill with fibromyalgia, I thought that if I just powered through my pain (like an athlete in training), the outcome would be positive. Hey, I was not going to give up! I was going to just try harder and harder to *ignore* the fact that it was painful even to walk up the stairs to my office each morning.

Lessons Learned:

One day I realized that instead of continuing to walk up the stairs every day (which resulted in ever-worsening leg and back pain) I would *accept* the fact that this activity, at this time, caused *unnecessary* pain. Therefore, it made sense to take the elevator and avoid the activity that caused me misery.

Reducing Symptoms Through Empowerment and Balance

Although there is currently no cure for fibromyalgia, there are many ways that you can manage the symptoms you experience. By becoming knowledgeable about your condition and accepting that it is a part of your life, you free yourself to look ahead, to consider various treatment options, and to find your way back to a happier, healthier, and more productive life. Knowledge and acceptance must also be coupled with empowerment and balance.

Empowerment comes from knowing that you have the ability to positively affect your own health. This does not mean that you can "cure" yourself with positive thoughts or by willing yourself to be well. It *does* mean that if you approach your illness with a healing attitude, you have a much better chance of improvement. You must learn which activities are good for your health and which ones are not, and then adjust your commitments accordingly.

If you view yourself as a sick person, you hinder your recovery. Accept your current reality so you can be more realistic with your expectations. But remember that reality can change, so continue to always remain open to pursue and try new things.

With all that I have learned throughout my journey with fibromyalgia, I believe that the key to improvement is finding balance. I strive to live a healthy life, both physically and emotionally. If you avoid extremes, you can become more balanced and things will probably become much easier. If you refuse to let go of preconceived ideas, such as "The harder I work, the more success I will have," you will miss the true keys to success: moderation and respecting your current limitations.

Picture This:

When I talk to people with fibromyalgia, I am always amazed by the adversity that they have overcome. Mary, an assembly-line worker who had never had any other type of job in her life, had the gumption to go through a job retraining program at age 55 to learn how to become a telephone operator. Jack and his wife restructured their whole life following his diagnosis; she became the breadwinner and he stayed at home with the kids. Maureen, who had to give up her dream of becoming a professional dancer, found tremendous happiness writing books about famous ballerinas. Debbie, who was haunted by her sleepless nights, began to paint when she couldn't sleep and established a business that produces watercolor greeting cards.

Lessons Learned:

No matter what obstacles are put before you, there are ways of getting around them. Your determination to overcome these challenges will empower you. Think of the individuals I mentioned above. Their willingness to find solutions to their life-altering challenges led to changing the direction of their lives—creating a new beginning.

Unlike the athlete who has to push through the pain, the person with fibromyalgia needs to nurture his or her body, listening to the signals it sends, and developing the discipline to obey those signals. Although all of us would like our recovery to be progressive, we must accept that the journey is not entirely straightforward. Sometimes we take one step forward and two steps back. Those down cycles are the most challenging, taunting us to succumb to negative thoughts and anger. With time, we can find the discipline to stay positive and get back on track. I speak with experience—the results of balance are worth the effort.

The following list shows you how to achieve balance.

How to Find Balance in Your Life

Learn to ...

- ◆ Make changes.
- ◆ Say no.
- ◆ Ask for help.
- ◆ Let yourself feel sad from time to time.
- ◆ Stop isolating yourself.

- Prioritize.

- Stop seeing a "friend" who is not understanding or supportive.

- Put your health first.

- Rest when you are tired.

- Change your mind if you need to.

- Be honest with yourself.

- Listen to your body.

- Disagree with your health-care professional and know that it's okay.

- Let a project go uncompleted if working on it makes your symptoms worse.

- Exercise gently.

- Simplify your life.

- Be realistic about your limitations.

- Be persistent as well as patient.

First Step: Acceptance

As discussed previously, to reduce your symptoms and take control of your health, you must first accept your illness. This does not mean that you are giving up hope for a symptom-free future. It just means that you must deal with the situation as it is now. You have to realize that you have a chronic disease and that you need discipline and patience to feel better. This section takes a closer look at some of the things you can do to develop acceptance.

Ten Goals for Accepting Your Illness

The following 10 goals will help you work through the process of *accepting your illness*. Each goal is followed by a series of questions to help you evaluate the different ways you can reach these goals. Note that the hints provided refer you to chapters in this book with additional information. Remember that the process of acceptance takes time and your feelings can vary day to day, month to month. Spend some time going through the following exercise and then repeat the process again after you have finished this book. You may find that you have moved closer to the goal of acceptance.

Goals Toward Acceptance

Goal 1: Get a proper diagnosis so you are certain that you have fibromyalgia.

Questions:

- Has your health-care professional performed a full medical history and tender-point exam on you in the last few months?

- If your doctor has not conducted a tender-point exam, what steps can you take to see a knowledgeable fibromyalgia health-care professional and get an examination that includes the accepted criteria for fibromyalgia diagnosis?

  Chapter 3 talks about who treats fibromyalgia and how you can find a good health-care professional who will perform a tender-point exam.

Goal 2: Know that fibromyalgia is not a progressive disease. Accept that your symptoms wax and wane. Symptom flares are transient and ultimately improve.

Questions:

- What can you do to deal with your illness when you have a symptom flare-up?

- What can you do to reduce the amount of stress you are experiencing when your symptoms are more prevalent?

- Where have you experienced improvement since you first became sick?

  Chapter 5 helps you to learn how to have a positive attitude and offers suggestions on ways to deal with stress.

Goal 3: Accept the fact that your life has to change, but know that this does not mean that your life cannot be full of happiness, self-fulfillment, and success.

Questions:

- What are the major changes that have occurred since you became sick?

- In what ways have these changes made your life better?

- If you still see certain changes as *bad*, what can you do to find better ways to deal with these changes?

- What new ways have you learned to make life easier or happier?

  For help in improving the way you look at the changes that have occurred in your life, see Chapter 5, which talks about steps toward better emotional well-being.

Goal 4: Don't do the things that irritate your symptoms, but find new ways to have fun and to participate in interesting and pleasurable activities.

Questions:

◆ What activities and situations make your symptoms worse?

◆ What can you do to avoid these activities and situations?

◆ What can you do to replace these activities and situations with others that are interesting and pleasurable?

Lifestyle changes are discussed in Chapter 8.

Goal 5: Take on a new experience. Doing so might fill you with trepidation, but taking risks and making changes often brings a new awareness of the joy of life experiences.

Questions:

◆ Can you list activities that are new to you, but add something positive to your life?

◆ What have you learned about yourself and others?

For help, read Chapter 8 for more information on lifestyle changes.

Goal 6: Don't constantly focus on what causes your symptoms to worsen or get better. Simple causes and effects can be difficult to identify in fibromyalgia. Concentrate instead on your self-management plan.

Questions:

◆ Have you stopped being analytical about everything that happens to you?

◆ Have you learned to accept that you will not always understand why some symptoms come and go?

Chapter 7 talks about the usefulness of biofeedback and cognitive behavioral therapy to help you focus your thoughts in a self-serving way.

Goal 7: Know that everyone with fibromyalgia is different. Don't compare your progress to that of others with the illness.

Question:

- What specifically have you done to ensure that you won't compare yourself to others?

  Chapter 7 discusses the reactions people have to each type of treatment and why fibromyalgia is treated with a multidisciplinary approach.

Goal 8: Eliminate your guilt and know that it is not your fault you have this illness.

Question:

- How have you reassured yourself that this illness is not your fault?

  For help, read Chapter 5 to learn about emotional well-being.

Goal 9: Incorporate a routine into your daily life. You should try a change, even if it does not sound like something you want to do. You might be surprised to find it is much easier than you expected.

Questions:

- What changes did you make that are now part of your daily routine?

- Even though you have done something one way for a long time, does that mean that it is the correct way to do it?

  Check out Chapter 8, which gives you ideas on how to simplify your life.

Goal 10: Let go of your fears and the "what ifs" and accept that life is different for you. Believe that it can still be wonderful.

Questions:

- Are you still afraid and unable to stop worrying about what things might be like in the future?

- Can you write out/express the way you want things to be and concentrate your thoughts on how you can make that future a reality?

  When you concentrate on the things you know, you take a positive step toward taking control of your future. Read more about how to do this in Chapter 5.

What Does Chronic Illness Mean to You?

Learning that you have a chronic illness can make you feel overwhelmed by thoughts of the future, and as if your life is out of control. There are things you can do to take back control and make the future seem less daunting. First, you have to know that the term *chronic illness* does not relate to a precise level of symptoms. A person can be chronically ill with a disease such as fibromyalgia and be significantly disabled, or a person can experience symptoms that are much less severe. While you will probably have this illness throughout your life, the level at which you will experience symptoms can and likely will vary greatly.

Taking responsibility for your illness gives you a sense of empowerment and increases your chances for improvement. This is why you should avoid focusing on the distant future. It is important for you to recognize that most experiences are limited and temporary. The majority of things we worry about never even happen. By worrying about the "what ifs," you are wasting valuable energy. Instead, try to take things one day at a time.

 Fast Fact

To increase your control over something that seems out of control, accept the situation for what it is and then implement RID:

- ◆ Redirect thoughts to the positive.
- ◆ Implement a balanced effort for change.
- ◆ Deal with the present.

What to Expect: The Stages of Acceptance

Change will become a part of your everyday routine. If you resist change, you resist the opportunity to improve your situation. It is important to remember that life is dynamic; what is true today may be different tomorrow. When you create your own personal self-management plan, you accept that your lifestyle will change (at least for now) and that change can be exciting and rewarding. For example, you might have always showered at night, but you realize that if you shower in the morning, the hot water eases sore muscles and reduces stiffness. The thought of changing this habit might not be pleasing, but after you implement the change and experience the benefits, you will become less resistant to this and other necessary changes.

If you have a bad day and focus on that, projecting it as the way things are going to be forever, you will be less able to cope successfully with the challenges ahead. If you understand that each day is different, you will feel more positive, realizing that tomorrow will probably be a far better day. Changes in your emotions and your approach will take you through the stages of acceptance and move you forward so that you can heal emotionally and physically. Each stage helps you learn about the healing process. The following list outlines the stages of acceptance, starting with the way you feel when you are first diagnosed.

When you feel that you have experienced and moved through a stage, check it off the list. You might skip a stage or go backward or forward through the stages.

The Ten Stages of Acceptance

1. **Uncertainty/Emotional Numbness.** When you're diagnosed with fibromyalgia, you may not understand what it means. You may feel relief because you have been searching for an explanation for your pain for a very long time. But when the reality sets in that you have an illness for which there is no cure, your reaction will probably be numbness and uncertainty.

2. **Processing.** When your health-care professional gives you a fibromyalgia diagnosis, he or she will probably give you some general background on the illness. The more information you get, the more questions you will have. Some of the answers will put your mind at ease; others will cause concern.

3. **Fear/Apprehension/Panic.** As you learn more about fibromyalgia and realize that you have been diagnosed with a chronic pain illness, your next response will probably be one of fear and apprehension. You will have countless questions. How will this affect your life? Will you get worse before you get better? How are you going to deal with this? As you start to think about the worst-case scenarios, you might panic or become overwhelmed.

4. **Frustration/Loss of Control.** At this stage, you will probably try to deny the diagnosis. You may feel very alone and search for the one health-care professional who can make you all better—fast. When this doesn't happen, you may feel frustrated and imagine that your life is spiraling out of control as the things you expect to happen ... don't. For example, you may think if you go to bed and rest for a day that you will feel fine—but you don't feel any better the next day. Or you will try to exercise to ease sore muscles, and instead you will hurt more the next day. This is the stage when you will discover that you are going to have to make changes to deal with fibromyalgia.

5. **Anger/Resentment.** When you realize that you are not going to be able to simply resume your former life, and you will have to make lifestyle changes, you may feel angry and resentful. You'll ask the following questions: Why did this

have to happen to me? What did I do to deserve this? You may feel resentment toward your health-care professional, family, or even God. Anger is a normal reaction, but it is not productive. You will be much better off when you channel your anger into more positive and healing emotions.

6. **Attempts to Resolve/Desire for Quick Resolution.** After you start letting go of your anger, you might find yourself trying to bargain your way out of this situation. Often an individual with fibromyalgia will try to resolve his or her illness by working to be a better person or making a deal with God. Sometimes a person with fibromyalgia wants to find a quick solution to his or her pain and will try products or attend seminars that promise a cure. This will usually lead to more frustration and wasted expenditures!

7. **Depression.** It is not unusual for a person with a chronic illness to become unhappy or even clinically depressed. Many studies have proven that fibromyalgia is not depression; however, depression can become one of the many symptoms of fibromyalgia. If you have always been a happy, positive person, this new symptom may seem very foreign and cause you much distress. The good news is that we understand depression much better today. We now know that depression is a chemical imbalance resulting in a range of symptoms. It is not something that you have to be embarrassed about or just put up with. And, fortunately, there are many ways to treat depression. Talk to your health-care professional about how you feel, and ask for a referral to a psychiatrist or psychologist who can help you deal with the many emotions and changes you experience.

8. **Reevaluation/New Focus.** As time progresses, you'll have the opportunity to become more educated about fibromyalgia and will start to realize that change is not so terrible after all; at this point, you will start the process of acceptance. You will reevaluate your life and realize that it is going to be different, but different does not have to be bad. You will start to find ways to improve your health and discover new opportunities that will become of interest to you. You will start to understand what "letting go" means. You will find that you don't have to *battle* against your illness, but rather can focus on a new lifestyle, a new purpose, and new interests.

9. **Recognition of the Situation.** As you move toward acceptance, you will become aware that there are many other people who share your same situation. You will learn that they experience the same challenges you do. Those who have a positive attitude, a good health-care professional or professionals, support from friends

and family, and the discipline to live life at a balanced pace experience improvement. You will find a new comfort with all the changes you have experienced. You will feel less fearful and more resolved to let go of the "what ifs." You will have a sense of calm about the future, and have faith that things will get better.

10. **Acceptance.** Acceptance does not mean resignation to a life of misery; it means you accept that things will be different. There are some things you can't control, but there are plenty of things you can. You will let go of the stressors and begin focusing on your priorities. You will learn how to manage the energy you have so that you don't exacerbate your symptoms. You may even start to see the benefits of having gone through this experience and recognize the positive results.

The Least You Need to Know

- After your fibromyalgia diagnosis, you learn to manage the illness.

- Accept your illness, learn ways to improve your quality of life, and discover that extraordinarily positive things can come out of an incredibly difficult experience.

- To reduce your symptoms and take control of your health, you must first accept your illness.

- Changes in your emotions and your approach will take you through the stages of acceptance and move you forward so that you can heal emotionally and physically.

Chapter 3

Develop and Implement a Self-Management Plan

In This Chapter

- ◆ Creating a self-management plan to improve your chances of enjoying better health
- ◆ Developing the seven steps of a self-management plan
- ◆ Evaluating "What Works Best for Me?"
- ◆ Implementing a self-management plan that helps you better understand your illness

When you have a broken leg, you go to the doctor and there is a protocol that exists for fixing the problem. When your leg is broken, you know there is something wrong and you know what the problem is. Your doctor can easily assess the situation, make a diagnosis, and treat the problem. Voilà! Problem solved. But there is a completely different scenario that exists when it comes to fibromyalgia.

First, fibromyalgia is polysymptomatic, in that it may express itself through many different symptoms, some of which you might not even recognize, such as sensitivity to light. When you go to a health-care professional with a long list of complaints, he will have to prioritize and evaluate your multiple symptoms in an efficient way. Fibromyalgia symptoms can mimic many diseases, and because there isn't a blood test or x-ray that can prove you have fibromyalgia, the first step is to rule out other diseases that might also present the same symptoms. Many health-care professionals are still learning about the diagnostic criteria and how to use them to diagnose fibromyalgia, so the process of "finding out what is wrong with you" often takes months and sometimes even years. And then after you know what is wrong, where do you begin? There is still much debate about an appropriate protocol for treating fibromyalgia, and to make matters even more confusing, everyone responds differently to treatment. For example, some people are helped by pharmacological interventions, yet others have a difficult time tolerating medicines. While some people respond more quickly to medical interventions, others need time to "adjust" to new treatment modalities and the process can be somewhat confusing.

So what do you do after you have been diagnosed with fibromyalgia? You develop your own individualized, time-tested self-management plan. You become educated about your options and then work toward finding the things that help reduce your symptoms.

Self-Management Steps

Now it is time to begin your journey to better health. First, recognize how important it is to develop your own personal self-management plan. Although you aren't alone in your efforts to reduce or eliminate symptoms, you are the captain of your team. This means that you must take an active role in your choices and efforts to improve your health. The steps discussed in the following sections guide you through the process of creating your own self-management plan. These steps include the following:

1. Educate yourself.

2. Gather opinions.

3. Listen to your body.

4. Analyze the options.

5. Set priorities.

6. Test through trial and error.

7. Narrow the field.

Picture This/Lessons Learned

Picture This:

When I first started to create my own personal self-management plan, I bought myself a bright pink (my favorite color) notebook that I used on a daily basis to jot down ideas, notes, and plans. When you start your own notebook, begin by writing 6 to 10 short sentences that outline how you plan to take charge of your own health care. Next, get creative. My notebook became a place where I could express my thoughts and ideas in any way I wanted. At one point I wrote a note to myself that expressed my desire to ride a bike again. Although it took years before I was able to accomplish this, writing it down planted the idea in my mind, and as I learned new ways to become more active, I found a way to get back on a bike!

Lessons Learned:

By writing things down, you organize your thoughts, allowing you to express your inner feelings, and even help discover new ways to deal with fibromyalgia. Your notebook will become a history of your experiences and goals, and will allow you to review what worked and what didn't. It will give you a better picture of how to become an expert at living with fibromyalgia.

Healthy Alternative

With each step, you will find suggestions for developing your own management plan. You might want to write down what you discover and learn as you move through the steps. Later you can use this information as a tool to help you develop your own personal plan.

Step 1: Educate Yourself

Knowledge and understanding reduce fears and assist you in learning what others have experienced and discovered.

Use the following resources to educate yourself:

♦ **Books.** These include books in print and on DVD!

♦ **Websites.** Make sure that you are "web wise" when you obtain information on the web. Check out Chapter 8 to learn more about evaluating the information you find on the Internet.

◆ **Local support groups.** Your local newspaper will often list upcoming community meetings on specific topics. Fibromyalgia support groups often meet at hospitals, libraries, churches, YMCAs, and other public places in your community.

◆ **National organizations.** Don't forget that I am the president of the National Fibromyalgia Association, and the organization is prepared to help you with additional information in preparation of your self-management plan (www. FMaware.org).

◆ **Newsletters.** There is an endless number of free newsletters on a wide range of topics.

◆ **Videos or DVDs.** Many organizations and universities are now developing informational videos that can be purchased for a minimal cost. Owning a video will allow you to watch and learn at your own pace.

◆ **Conferences.** National organizations host annual scientific meetings that present the latest research and offer specialized educational opportunities in the field of multidisciplinary pain management. Programs are often designed for a particular audience; however, many are appropriate for both physicians and patients.

◆ **Medical journals.** There are numerous medical journals that present scientific abstracts on the diagnosis and treatment of fibromyalgia and overlapping conditions.

◆ **Blogs.** Personal websites that are made publicly accessible in order to share an individual's opinions and views. Although these sites are not monitored for accuracy, they can provide information on fibromyalgia that might be useful.

◆ **Blogtalkradio.com.** A web-based platform that enables any individual to host a live blog show online. The service is free for blog show hosts and listeners. The National Fibromyalgia Association hosts a show on a monthly basis.

◆ **Podcasts.** Audio broadcasts that are made available on the web and can be downloaded to a computer or audio player. Podcast.net has a directory of fibromyalgia broadcasts.

◆ **Online chats.** Find the chat room that fits with your philosophies and where the members remain optimistic and helpful.

◆ **Federal government clearinghouses.** You can start with the National Institutes of Health at www.nih.gov.

- ◆ **Medical, hospital, or university libraries.** Call your local hospital to find out whether it hosts a fibromyalgia support group or has brochures or informational packets on the subject. If you are looking for specific medical information, you might be able to find it at a university library.

- ◆ **Nurse, pharmacy, or other health help lines and directories.** Talking to pharmacists or a nurse at your health-care provider's office might give you answers to questions that you weren't able to talk to your doctor about. Call your local Chamber of Commerce and ask whether there is a directory that lists social services and medical agencies available in your community.

- ◆ **Health-insurance company question-and-answer telephone lines.** Some insurance companies have 800 numbers for health-help lines available to their patients, 24 hours a day. Prerecorded information can provide you with valuable facts and resources. Ask your insurance carrier whether it has a directory that lists all the services its help line offers. Some companies actually have a counselor or health-care professional available to speak to you directly.

For more information on where to find these types of reference materials, refer to Appendix B.

 Pain Signal _____

Remember that we live in a world of vast amounts of information. Not all information is accurate or helpful. When researching information, don't forget to use information wisely. Ask yourself the following questions:

- ◆ Is this a credible source?
- ◆ Is this source trying to sell me something?
- ◆ When applying common sense, does this information make sense?
- ◆ What do other resources say? Is the information similar?
- ◆ Are references listed for the information?

Step 2: Gather Opinions

Part of discovering and understanding your illness is talking to a variety of people. You won't always agree with everything you hear, but it will help you determine what ideas and concepts you are comfortable with. I suggest that you collect the opinion of the following individuals:

- Medical health-care professionals
- Complementary health-care specialists
- Support-group leaders
- Members of a support group
- Family members
- Friends who have gone through life-challenging situations
- Religious leaders
- Web message boards and chats

Step 3: Listen to Your Body

You can learn a lot by becoming more aware of the signals that your body sends you. Pay attention to the following statements, and if you experience these feelings often, you should share this information with your health-care professional:

- You feel unhappy or blue.
- You wake up unrefreshed and tired.
- You feel a tingling sensation in various parts of your body.
- Your neck and shoulders are tense and feel like they are in knots.
- You feel out of breath.
- You have a hard time concentrating or remembering.
- You wake up multiple times throughout the night.
- Bright lights or certain smells seem excessively intense.
- You feel achy and notice pain all over your body.
- Your energy level seems exceptionally low.
- You get night sweats and often feel feverish.
- You have more pain when the weather changes.
- You notice that you have less patience than usual.
- Your body hurts after you do minimal amounts of exercise.
- At night your legs twitch and you get muscle cramps.

- You are tired during the day and awake at night.

- You become constipated or often have diarrhea.

- You get headaches or migraines.

- Your mouth and eyes are exceptionally dry.

- Your hands are sensitive to cold and your fingers turn blue.

Step 4: Analyze What Works Best for You

Because fibromyalgia is treated with multiple treatment options, you have to evaluate the options you feel the most comfortable with. Usually it is helpful to base this analysis on things that have worked well for you in the past. (But do not be afraid to try new things.)

Following is a list of multiple treatment options that you might want to consider:

Western Medicine

Pharmaceuticals

Narcotics for pain

Physical therapy

Exercise

Alternative Medicine

Supplements

Herbs

Acupuncture

Massage

Chiropractic manipulation

Yoga, Tai Chi, etc.

Aquatic therapy

Nutrition or diet changes

Homeopathy

Counseling

Psychotherapy

Cognitive behavior therapy

Biofeedback

Hypnosis

Attending a support group

Unproven or Experimental Treatments

Participate in clinical trials

Step 5: Set Priorities

It is important to try different treatments one at a time so you know what effect each treatment produces. (Keep in mind, however, that because your emotions affect your physical condition, it is important to deal with emotional issues as soon as possible.)

The following list will help familiarize you with the specialists and treatment options available to you. Review the list, and then check off the health-care professionals that you *think* you would like to see and the treatment options you *think* you would like to try, based on your beliefs and personal needs. As you progress through this book, you will learn more about the health-care professionals and the treatment options that are available to you. You will want to refine your choices as you move forward in the development of your self-management plan.

Health-Care Professionals

- Family practice health-care professional
- Internist/rheumatologist
- Pain-management specialist
- Neurologist
- Osteopath
- Neuropath
- Counselor
- Psychologist

- Psychiatrist
- Social worker
- Occupational therapist
- Physical therapist
- Nutritional specialist

    Chapter 4 provides you with specific information on health-care providers.

Treatment Options

- Pharmaceuticals
- Narcotics for pain
- Antidepressants for pain/sleep
- Antidepressants for depression
- Analgesics for pain
- Sleep medication
- Anti-inflammatories for pain
- Anti-anxiety medication
- Cognitive behavior therapy
- Biofeedback
- Acupuncture
- Massage
- Chiropractic
- Homeopathy
- Aquatic therapy
- Yoga or Pilates
- Hypnosis
- Guided imagery
- Meditation

- Supplements

- Herbs

- Group therapy or support group

- Unproven or experimental treatments

- Other

  Chapters 9 and 10 will provide you with specific information about treatment options.

Step 6: Test Through Trial and Error

Every person with fibromyalgia reacts differently to the treatments they try. Some treatments result in side effects that are too severe to put up with, whereas others might have side effects that last only a short period of time. Many things you try will have a positive effect on your symptoms, and some might have no effect at all.

Fast Fact

A "side effect" can show intolerance to a certain type of medication or treatment; however, it can also be a temporary reaction while your body adjusts to something new. Talk to your health-care provider for more information.

Remember that people with fibromyalgia are often sensitive to medications, and it is smart to talk to your health-care professional about starting on a smaller-than-normal dosage. It is important to work with your health-care professional or alternative-care practitioner to evaluate the success of a treatment and determine whether you need to abandon it and try something else. It is also important to have patience when trying a variety of medications or alternative treatments before finding the ones that are right for you.

Step 7: Narrow the Field

As you develop your self-management plan, prioritize the options you want to try first. It is important to start with options that have been proven to be successful for the majority of people with fibromyalgia. Because you don't want to try too many things at one time, start by dealing with your emotions and how you are going to live with this illness (see Chapter 14). Then try the treatment options that are most effective (see Chapter 9). Finally you can add options that are not clinically proven for fibromyalgia patients, but that have been helpful to some.

Refining Your Self-Management Plan

Now that you have begun to accept your illness, become more educated, talked to experts, learned how to listen to your body, and evaluated treatment plans and options, you should have the tools to proceed in the right direction. You have set goals and evaluated and prioritized treatment options, and now it is time to put these individual thoughts into an action plan.

Remember that you are setting out on a journey that will be made up of bumps and smooth patches, twists and turns, and straight-aways. You are in charge of your plan, but it will be easier to implement it if you create a team to help you put your plan into action. These important people in your life will influence your decisions and they will offer you support.

How to Deal With Waxing and Waning

Fibromyalgia is a disease that waxes and wanes, or in other words, gets worse and then better and continues in this pattern for a long period of time. It is important to know that the span of time that passes between highs and lows will become longer and the intensity of the highs and lows will decrease over time. If you realize that the bad times are not going to be permanent and you find ways to treat the more difficult symptoms, you will feel in control and less frustrated with the down times.

For example, when you first get sick, you might have many overlapping conditions and you will want to see health-care professionals who can help you with these symptoms. (Chapter 1 lists these conditions.) If you get migraine headaches or restless legs under control, your overall symptoms will improve and the waxing and waning of fibromyalgia symptoms will not happen as frequently or as intensely.

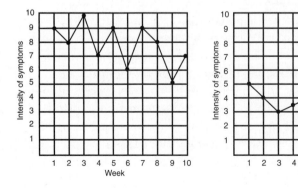

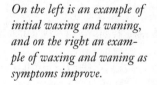

On the left is an example of initial waxing and waning, and on the right an example of waxing and waning as symptoms improve.

Keeping to a Daily Routine

Because fibromyalgia symptoms are affected by even the slightest changes or influences on your nervous system (for example, changes in sleep, eating habits, noises, hormone changes, or workload), it is helpful to keep to a daily routine, allowing your body to "balance itself" and avoid stressors. This means changing your lifestyle, but you will notice the positive effects it will have on your symptoms.

The following list gives examples of how to establish a routine:

◆ Go to bed and get up at the same time every day.

◆ Eat three to four small meals daily—at the same time every day.

◆ Schedule rest times when you lie down in a quiet, comfortable place three times a day for 10 to 15 minutes.

◆ Make changes to your environment that will eliminate harsh lights, loud noises, and variations in temperature.

◆ Have a family member or a friend help you rearrange your house so that items are more accessible.

◆ Arrange a time each day to do something that makes you happy.

Appreciating Successes

Because your quality of life will improve slowly over time, you might not always recognize the gradual improvements. Even though your pain is less, you might still be frustrated by the level of pain you are experiencing. It is important to recognize and appreciate the improvements you *do* experience. Every month, make a note of the improvements you have seen. Mentally take note of the improvements and focus on them. If you actually create a mental picture of you doing the activity, it will help the image stand out in your memory. I have vivid pictures in my mind of specific activities that I did for the first time after I got sick. The first time I walked to the mailbox, the first time I completed a water therapy class, the first time I got on an airplane and went somewhere, the first time I got on a treadmill … and thousands more!

The Least You Need to Know

♦ Review the seven steps for developing a self-management plan, and create your own self-management plan.

♦ There are multiple treatment options that work to varying degrees for different people. An analysis of these options will help you to decide what options you want to include in your own self-management plan.

♦ Although fibromyalgia waxes and wanes over time, by developing your own personal self-management plan you will increase the amount of time between having only a few symptoms and having your symptoms worsen.

♦ When implementing your self-management plan, it is helpful if you keep to a daily routine, allowing your body to "balance itself."

♦ Be sure to recognize the improvements that you experience. Even if they are small improvements, take note.

Part **2**

Who Can Help Me?

The old adage "two heads are better than one" rings true when it comes to fibromyalgia. Finding the right individuals to give you support and to provide the necessary medical expertise will ensure that you have an advantage when it comes to improving your health. Finding a balance between taking responsibility for your own health and also trusting in others who will become a part of your health-care team is vital. Learning when and how to ask for help will encourage others to be there when you need them.

You must remember that your illness affects everyone around you. It is important that you are sensitive to their needs, too, and by working together you will find ways to modify and improve the many aspects of your family's life that may have changed. Good communication and the willingness to compromise will help everyone adjust and eventually feel comfortable with these new challenges.

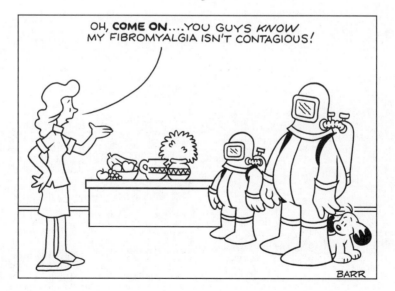

Assembling Your Health-Care Team

In This Chapter

- ◆ Having two heads is better than one
- ◆ Taking charge of your health-care team
- ◆ Choosing medical specialists for your team
- ◆ Finding a doctor
- ◆ Winning your family's support
- ◆ Adding a pet to your health-care team

Today, not only is the idea of physician and patient collaboration more common than ever before, it has been shown to increase the likelihood that a patient will improve over time. The trend of a patient participating in their own health-care decisions makes even more sense when it comes to fibromyalgia, because patients differ in symptomology and response to treatment. For the fibromyalgia patient who has become informed about their medical options, is in tune with the messages that their body sends them, and has created a partnership through open and truthful communication with their health-care providers, they are almost guaranteed improvement in their quality of life.

Your health-care team may have a variety of participants, such as a family member who goes with you to your doctor appointments, a massage therapist or yoga instructor who is concerned about specific complementary treatment, and of course your medical heath-care provider. The key, however, is when a patient and their doctor become a collaborative team, each playing an important role in the process of "treatment." The physician can provide information and motivation, and even challenge their patient to do what they feel is medically effective. However, ultimately it's up to the patient to decide to accept or reject the advice of the physician and implement the recommended plan for treatment. In many situations you will be making important decisions based on the information you have collected, and ultimately it will be up to you to carry out the various elements of the plan on your own.

It is important that patients recognize the importance of asking their physicians questions regarding medical tests, diagnoses, and medications. If a patient feels empowered to ask questions, such as what specific tests will determine, why certain medications are being prescribed, and what expectations they should have for the future, they will be more competent in making important medical decisions.

Assembling and Captaining Your Team

The old adage "two heads are better than one" highlights the power of collaboration. In a challenging situation, discussing issues with others, listening to others' ideas, and weighing others' suggestions is extremely helpful and usually produces a better end result. Assembling a health-care team enables you to draw on many individuals' strengths, knowledge, and support.

Fast Fact _____

You may be surprised about who can be a helpful team member. The office manager in your doctor's office may be able to keep you informed about your medical paperwork, and the little girl next door may be helpful in taking care of your pets and bringing you your mail. Don't rule out anyone who could have an interest in helping you!

The ideal group to support a person with fibromyalgia consists of diverse people: health-care professionals, family, friends, support group members, organizations, and others who can empower the patient. As the captain of your team, you need to be sure everyone is focused on the same goal—helping _you_ improve your health. Your task is to match prospective team members' skills with the different needs you have, so each member can play a unique and vital role in your health care.

It is essential that you trust your team members (especially the health-care professionals) and that everyone listens with an open mind to the suggestions of the other members (especially you). For example, if your husband thinks your physician is not reliable—and you and your doctor feel that trying a new medication is important—your husband may not be supportive of that treatment option.

Do not hesitate to add to or change the members of your team. These individuals must be committed to supporting and helping *you* get healthier. If any member of the team increases your stress level or does not respect your needs, you should communicate your concerns. Remember that this team is not an official, organized unit (unless you have multiple medical specialists who are consulting together on your case), but rather a group of individuals you know and trust and believe can assist you. Over time your team may change; one-time members may eventually take no part in your care, while others may join with new ideas and options.

Taking Charge of Your Illness

It may seem obvious, but it is important to remember that you are the most important person on your health-care team. You set the tone and direction of the group, and have the most influence over the outcome. It is vital to keep this in mind, because it gives you back some control in a situation that may have made you feel powerless. You need to rely on others' opinions, but ultimately you make the decisions.

Picture This/Lessons Learned

Picture This:

As you develop your health-care team, be sure that your expectations are fair. Some people will help you and expect nothing in return (except maybe your gratitude); however, there will be members who expect to be compensated for their assistance because it is their *job* to provide you with certain services for a fee.

A friend of mine used to come over quite often and bring me homemade soup or a casserole that she had made. I very much appreciated her efforts and thanked her often. As time went on she started to come by less often and I missed her friendship. When I finally got up the courage to ask her why she wasn't coming over anymore, she explained that it got expensive covering the cost of the food she was bringing me. I hadn't realized that this was a hardship for her and quickly let her know that I had no problem reimbursing her for the cost of the food!

Lessons Learned:

Having fibromyalgia isn't fair, and you may feel like you therefore *deserve* things from people—but it is important to remain appreciative and open to paying for professional services. If you were providing a service, wouldn't you expect to be paid for your expertise?

By the time I finally accepted my illness and realized that I had to decide who would be part of my health-care team, I was suffering from a lack of confidence. The difficulties I'd experienced in getting a diagnosis, and the realization that I was vulnerable to a chronic illness, had left me unable to trust my decision-making ability. I was desperately afraid that if I asked someone to help me, they might actually make me worse!

For example, one friend told me: "All you need is to join a gym with me, and we will exercise you right back to health." Instead, after visiting the sports center twice, I ended up $100 poorer, feeling worse than I had before exercising.

Pain Signal _____

Self-confidence is believing in and acting on your actions and decisions. Chronic illness can change your abilities, so you must learn to live with a new set of abilities and truths about yourself. It might take some time to rebuild your self-confidence, but it is important to strive to do so.

It is not unusual to experience feelings of inadequacy and to question your ability to make good decisions when your life has been changed by fibromyalgia. However, it is important to realize that the only way to get your self-confidence back is by forming a health-care team to advise you, and then to base your decisions on their informed and reliable suggestions. My girlfriend was great at advising me on how to rearrange my house so that it would be more "fibro-friendly," but when it came to exercise, I should have asked someone knowledgeable on the subject, such as my doctor or a physical therapist.

Building a team might also seem foreign to you, especially if you have always preferred going it alone. Maybe you fear that asking for help will appear to be a sign of weakness. Put this thought out of your head! Everyone needs help from time to time—and this is your time. Remember even the most powerful and successful people in the world, such as a president, CEO, or world-class athlete, have advisors, mentors, and coaches. Everyone benefits when there are "two heads" instead of one!

What happens, however, if you are alone (not by choice)? Maybe you aren't married or you do not have family members living near you. What if you feel truly all alone?

Never fear. You can find many different people to join your health-care team: medical professionals, clergy, neighbors, Internet contacts, support group members, and so on. When you start to make a list of those people who could become a part of your team, you will discover that you are not alone at this time. Do not ever be afraid, embarrassed, or hesitant to ask for help, voice your opinion, or seek the care you need and deserve.

To help you select members of your health-care team, go to Appendix C and fill out the chart labeled "Your Health-Care Team." As you find members to add to your team, be sure to log their contact information so they will always be easy to contact.

Who Treats Fibromyalgia?

When you first experience fibromyalgia symptoms, you might seek the help of a family physician, internist, OB-GYN, gastroenterologist, or psychologist. Some of these clinicians are knowledgeable about fibromyalgia and may evaluate your symptoms based on the criteria for diagnosis.

In the past, people with fibromyalgia or its symptoms (especially body-wide pain, fatigue, sleep disturbances, and cognitive difficulties) sought the opinion of a qualified rheumatologist. A *rheumatologist* is an internist or pediatrician who has received an additional two to three years of training and experience in the diagnosis and treatment of arthritis and other diseases of the joints, muscles, and bones. Because of their experience in treating musculoskeletal pain disorders, rheumatologists were the group of doctors most knowledgeable about and willing to treat fibromyalgia.

In recent years, awareness and knowledge of fibromyalgia has grown dramatically. Now it is not uncommon for people with the symptoms of fibromyalgia to discover that their family practice doctors are familiar with the illness, its diagnosis, and the treatment spectrum. The American Academy of Family Physicians is working hard to ensure that its members are well educated about fibromyalgia, and Continuing Medical Education programs about fibromyalgia are in development for family physicians.

 Pain Signal

Watch for red flags—for example, when people make extravagant claims that they can "cure" you, or use testimonials that work on your emotions but go against common sense. If it seems too good to be true, it probably is! Be sure that you do research and bring only credible individuals to your team.

 Fast Fact

The American College of Rheumatology believes that seeking out the care of a rheumatologist may save time and money and reduce the severity of fibromyalgia symptoms. By seeing a specially trained rheumatologist (one who is well versed in the diagnosis and treatment of fibromyalgia), you can ensure that the proper tests are done early—and you might even save money in the long run. An accurate, prompt diagnosis and specially tailored treatment program will increase your chances of quick symptom improvement.

As medical professionals continue to become better educated about fibromyalgia, it is more and more often the case that patients can turn to their primary care providers for answers and support.

Medical Professionals (Specialties)

You are likely to have a lead health-care team member (whether that person is a rheumatologist or your primary care provider), but this doctor is likely to be only a part of your medical professional team. If you experience overlapping conditions such as migraine headaches, restless legs syndrome, or irritable bowel syndrome, you may want to consult with other specialists.

Following is a list of several health-care team member options. These are only options! Each patient's situation is unique, and will require a different set of health-care experts. Carefully consider who may best help you manage your specific situation and symptom set. You may also want to refer back to Chapter 3 and review Step 5 of the self-management program (where you ranked the medical professionals you feel most comfortable talking to).

- ◆ **Family practice physician.** A family practice physician offers general medical care to people of all ages. Ongoing care includes preventive health care, as well as care for acute and chronic illness of all kinds, including fibromyalgia. A growing number of family practice physicians have a strong interest in and knowledge of fibromyalgia.

- ◆ **Neurologist.** A neurologist is a board-certified medical doctor trained in the diagnosis and treatment of nervous system disorders, including diseases of the brain, spinal cord, nerves, and muscles. A neurologist performs examinations of the nerves of the body; muscle strength, movement, and reflexes; balance and ambulation; and sensation, memory, speech, language, and other cognitive abilities. A neurologist also treats headaches, migraines, and restless legs syndrome.

- ◆ **Gastroenterologist.** A gastroenterologist is an internist who specializes in the diagnosis and treatment of diseases of the digestive organs, including the stomach, bowels, liver, and gallbladder. This specialist treats conditions such as abdominal pain, ulcers, diarrhea and constipation, irritable bowel syndrome, and autoimmune diseases of the gut.

- ◆ **Doctor of osteopathy.** A doctor of osteopathy (D.O.) completes the same amount of medical education as an M.D. and must pass a state licensing examination. A D.O. can perform surgery, treat patients, and prescribe medications in both clinic and hospital settings. A D.O. is trained to perform osteopathic manipulations, a technique in which the D.O. uses the hands to diagnose illness and treat patients, giving special attention to the joints, bones, muscles, and nerves.

♦ **Allergist-immunologist.** An allergist-immunologist is trained in evaluating and managing disorders involving the immune system. Examples of such conditions include asthma, rhinitis, eczema, and adverse reactions to drugs, foods, and insect stings, as well as immune-deficiency diseases.

♦ **Pain-management specialist.** A pain-management specialist is an anesthesiologist, neurologist, pediatric neurologist, physiatrist, or psychologist who provides a high level of care, either as a primary physician or consultant, for patients experiencing problems with acute and chronic pain (including cancer pain).

♦ **Physiatrist.** A physiatrist is an M.D. specializing in physical medicine and rehabilitation who treats a wide range of problems from sore shoulders to spinal cord injuries. Those who specialize in physiatry focus on restoring functions.

Other Health-Care Professionals

Remember that health-care professionals who are not medical doctors can also play an important role on your health-care team.

♦ **Pharmacist.** A pharmacist can assist you with questions about your prescriptions, drug interactions, and side effects. A *compounding pharmacist* goes beyond dispensing manufactured drugs.

def•i•ni•tion

Some patients are not good candidates for mass-produced drugs. They may be allergic to preservatives or dyes in the drugs, or be sensitive to standard drug strengths. In these cases, a **compounding pharmacist** can prepare a drug to alter its strength, eliminate the allergens, or make it more digestible or palatable.

♦ **Nurse.** Nurses are an extremely important part of your health-care team. Nurses have a wide range of skills and are usually in charge of implementing the care your doctor has set up for you. They are trained to administer medication and monitor side effects. Nurses are often aware of support services in your community and can usually provide you with educational materials and pamphlets.

◆ **Physical therapist.** A physical therapist provides patients with services that help them restore function, improve mobility, and relieve pain, and can assist and help promote overall health fitness. Working closely with a physiatrist, a physical therapist employs such modalities as stretching, muscle strengthening, range-of-motion exercises, heat/ice, electrical stimulation, ultrasound, traction, and mobilization. A physical therapist tests and measures the patient's strength, range of motion, balance and coordination, posture, muscle performance, respiration, and motor function.

◆ **Registered dietitian.** A registered dietitian must meet the rigorous academic requirements of the Commission on Dietetic Registration, and can assist you with your nutrition or food preparation/service needs.

◆ **Acupuncturist.** The requirements to practice *acupuncture* vary significantly worldwide. To legally practice acupuncture in Europe, a practitioner must first be a medical doctor. In the United States, nonphysicians may be licensed to practice acupuncture. Acupuncture is commonly used to help ease headaches, arthritis, back and neck pain, soreness, nausea, sinus pain, insomnia, PMS or painful cramps, and a wide variety of other conditions. It is also effective in reducing stress and helping one to make constructive lifestyle changes.

def•i•ni•tion

Acupuncture involves therapeutic needles being placed in various combinations and patterns all over the body. The acupuncturist inserts the needles in patterns that are based on the traditional principle of encouraging the flow of qi (pronounced "chee"), a subtle energy that flows through acupuncture channels.

◆ **Massage therapist.** A massage therapist is a professional practitioner who applies a series of manual therapeutic soft-tissue manipulations by applying pressure to the body.

◆ **Aquatic therapist.** An aquatic therapist specializes in a variety of aquatic techniques that allow the patient to move in a water environment. The buoyancy of the water allows the patient to perform low-impact exercises without stressing the muscles and joints. Many people can perform exercises in water that they cannot do out of the water. Specialty aquatic techniques include …

Ai Chi—A form of active aquatic therapy modeled after the principles of Tai Chi and yoga breathing techniques.

Watsu—A form of passive aquatic therapy performed in a hands-on manner by the provider. The client is usually held or cradled in warm water while the provider stabilizes or moves one part of the person's body, resulting in the stretching of another part of the body due to the drag effect.

♦ **Occupational therapist.** An occupational therapy practitioner is a professional whose education includes the study of human growth and development with an emphasis on the social, emotional, and physiological effects of illness and injury. An occupational therapist evaluates all facets of the client's life to help that person find the skills for the job of living. Treatment programs are customized specifically to help the client perform daily activities and give guidance to the client's family members.

Emotional Health-Care Professionals

Health-care professionals who specialize in mental health will ensure that your emotional needs are also being met. Even if you aren't dealing with depression or another mental health issue, people who are faced with lifestyle changes and chronic pain can often benefit from the care of this type of specialist:

♦ **Psychologist.** A psychologist is a Ph.D. who provides therapy and counseling if you are feeling sad, depressed, anxious, or stressed out. Moreover, a psychologist can help you cope with pain by using cognitive behavioral therapy. Although not medical doctors, psychologists have a doctoral degree in psychology and counseling and may specialize in marital counseling or chronic illness.

♦ **Psychiatrist.** A psychiatrist is a medical doctor who specializes in diagnosing and treating mental, addictive, and emotional disorders. These doctors specialize in treating mood disorders, anxiety disorders, schizophrenia, and adjustment disorders. The psychiatrist is able to understand the biological, psychological, and social components of these illnesses, and treats the person as a whole. A psychiatrist can order diagnostic laboratory tests, prescribe medications, evaluate and treat psychological and interpersonal problems, and assist families who are coping with stress, crises, and other problems.

♦ **Social worker.** A social worker is professionally trained in counseling and practical assistance. A clinical or psychiatric social worker has an advanced degree or a Ph.D. and is trained to provide family therapy, marital counseling, or counseling about coping with chronic illness. A local hospital social worker can refer you to a clinical social worker in private practice in your community.

◆ **Clergy.** Prayer and spiritual counseling can be very important in coping with a serious illness. Many people find it useful to get help from clergy or other spiritual leaders. Even if your beliefs are challenged by your illness, don't be afraid to reach out for help.

Finding a Health-Care Professional Who Is Right for You

Now that you know there are many qualified health-care professionals to choose from, how do you find the right ones for you? Having an M.D. does not automatically make a clinician a good doctor for *you*. It is important to check the professional's credentials, interview him, and see whether you feel you can successfully create a partnership. If you were going to hire a babysitter or attorney, you would always want to know specific information about that person. Likewise, there are certain questions you are going to want to ask of health-care professionals before engaging their services. Each patient has unique requirements of a doctor. It is important that you give your requirements a great deal of thought.

Guide to Finding a Doctor

Following is a list of requirements related to finding the right doctor for you. Rate each one on a scale of 1 to 5, with 5 being essential and 1 being not very important. When you interview or evaluate a potential doctor, be sure that person meets all requirements that you rank as a 4 or higher.

_____ Geographic location/office hours

_____ Treats other people with fibromyalgia

_____ Types of insurance accepted

_____ Costs

_____ Willing to spend time with you

_____ Treatment philosophy—aggressive/conservative

_____ Looks at you as an equal, not as your boss

_____ Types of treatments offered

_____ Good bedside manner

_____ Believes what you say and listens to your concerns

_____ Is willing to explain things, including medical terms, purpose of medications, and side effects

_____ Helps with referrals and communicating with other physicians

_____ Is open-minded to alternative and complementary treatments

_____ Is willing to talk to your family and help them to be supportive

---

Healthy Alternative

To avoid any potential problems, be sure that your doctor was trained at a reputable institution and has a valid medical license. Without a medical license, a doctor is not legally allowed to treat patients. To verify a medical license in your state, you can contact the Federation of State Medical Boards at 817-868-4000.

If you are interested in seeing a specialist, be sure that you find one who is board certified. Although a board certification is not legally necessary to practice medicine, a physician who is board certified is more likely to have additional medical knowledge. A board-certified physician must successfully complete an approved educational program, complete an evaluation process, and pass an exam. The certification is valid nationwide. To find out if a particular physician is board certified, you can call the American Board of Medical Specialties (ABMS) toll-free: 1-866-ASK-AMBS.

Resources for Finding a Doctor

Now that you know what you want and need from a doctor, you must find a group of doctors to consider. There are numerous ways to do this.

First, ask your friends, family, and neighbors if they have a physician they highly recommend. (Be careful! Not everyone likes the same kind of doctor.) Check online for medical or fibromyalgia organizations that have doctor referral lists. You can also talk to a local fibromyalgia support group, which should be able to give you the names of physicians that its members see. Here are some organizations you may want to check:

National Fibromyalgia Association
714-921-0150
www.FMaware.org

Arthritis Foundation
www.arthritis.org

American College of Rheumatology
Members Directory:
www.rheumatology.org/directory/geo.asp

HealthGrades
www.healthgrades.com/consumer/index.
cfm?fuseaction=homepage&tv_eng=Google&tvkw=C3AG8

American Medical Association
www.ama-assn.org/ama/pub/category/9858.html

Fast Fact _____

A smart way to find a good physician is to identify the best hospitals in your community (the best hospitals usually attract the best doctors).

American Academy of Medical Acupuncture
www.medicalacupuncture.org/findadoc/index.html

American Academy of Pain Management
www.aapainmanage.org/search/MemberSearch.php

Doctors for Pain.com
www.doctorsforpain.com/physicians/index.html

Med Help.com
www.med-help.net/Fibromyalgia-Doctors.html

You can also call your health insurance company, which can send you a directory of physicians who accept your insurance plan. And finally, talk to your current doctor and ask whether he or she can recommend a doctor in the specialty area that you are interested in.

After you have a list of referred physicians, contact their offices and speak to the office personnel or ask to meet or talk to the physician. Remember, it is not unusual to interview a doctor before choosing to accept treatment from him or her.

How to Win the Support of Family and Friends

One of the challenges of fibromyalgia is that you don't look sick. Family and friends might have a hard time accepting your illness because it is not visibly obvious to them. Because fibromyalgia is a condition that waxes and wanes, it can be difficult to understand why you are able to do some things one day and not the next. Therefore, you will need to make every possible effort to help educate your loved ones, and to communicate the reality of your situation to those who are part of your life.

Take into account that your "invisible" illness is going to have an impact on the people in your life—especially your immediate family. *Together* you need to understand what it means to have fibromyalgia—that it is no one's fault, and that by working together and dealing with the problems and creating solutions, everyone will benefit in the future.

One of the most important things you can do is to recognize that fibromyalgia is changing the lives of your friends and family, too. Even though you might feel that all the attention should be on *you* and helping *you* to get better, consider what your loved ones are going through. Imagine your family's feelings of frustration, worry, and fear. Just like you, they need to understand this disease, to feel some control over it, and to know they can become a part of the solution. Some family members may choose to ignore the problem, because then they do not have to deal with it. But just like you, your family needs to accept the situation for what it is right now and find ways to communicate and work together to improve things for everyone.

Picture This/Lessons Learned

Picture This:

Olivia's recent diagnosis of fibromyalgia has put her at odds with her husband, William. She feels he is always angry because of her inability to do the things they used to do together. William can't understand why all of a sudden his wife has become withdrawn and has no interest in activities they used to enjoy together.

Lessons Learned:

The truth is that Olivia feels like she has let her husband down by becoming ill, and she is uncomfortable trying to explain to him that she feels both guilty and fearful. William is not angry with his wife; he is concerned about her and feels hurt that it seems she no longer wants to do things with him. He doesn't understand that it is her illness keeping her from doing the activities they used to enjoy together. Improved communication will help both Olivia and William realize that they aren't mad at each other. From there, they can work together to come up with new activities they can enjoy together.

In order for your loved ones to become health-care team members, they must become educated about fibromyalgia; accept that your symptoms are very real; be aware that you are striving to improve your quality of life; and understand that their support can be a major factor in your chances of getting better.

Be truthful with your family members. If they see that you are actively working toward implementing a self-management plan, that you communicate your level of pain and fatigue (not only when it is bad, but also when it is good), and that you support them with the issues they are facing, you will find yourself in a cooperative situation: everyone is working toward the same goal—to help you get better.

Healthy Alternative

Family members should be assured that you don't expect them to have all the answers. Be sure they understand how much it helps if they just listen to how you feel and let you know they hear you.

A third party can play an important role in educating your loved ones about the reality of life with fibromyalgia. Many people with fibromyalgia find it worthwhile to have their spouse or significant other attend their doctor's appointments, support group meetings, or family and marital counseling sessions. Communication is the key. Do not be afraid to be truthful with one another. Be respectful of each other's situations. Become *jointly* committed to the process of improvement.

Pets and Your Health

Have you considered adding a pet (or two) to your health-care team? According to the National Institutes of Health (NIH), studies have shown that the bonds people form with pets can help improve certain health conditions. Pets make wonderful companions and can bring you happiness and unconditional love. Dogs are always eager to help you with your exercise program, cats never talk back, and even a bird can sing you a song, lift your spirits, and make you smile. If a pet can help improve your health, it will make a valuable contribution to the team.

The Least You Need to Know

- Assemble a health-care team and utilize the combined strengths, knowledge, and support of the team members.

- Do not hesitate to ask for help, voice your opinion, or seek the care you need and deserve. You must become an active member of your team, promoting open communication.

- Numerous health-care professionals with varying perspectives and a wide range of specialized knowledge can become important contributors to your heath-care team.

- Research a physician before you decide to add him or her to your health-care team. As you would with any other expert you hire to help you, check potential health-care providers' credentials.

- Recognize that fibromyalgia also changes the lives of family members.

- Pets make great health-care team members. They give unconditional love and are always willing to listen!

Communication and Relationships

In This Chapter

- ◆ Communicating well is important
- ◆ Learning that what you say is as important as how you say it
- ◆ Overcoming obstacles to create good communication
- ◆ Talking about your fibromyalgia
- ◆ Improving your family's communication

I remember getting a Princess telephone for my sixteenth birthday. Talking on it was my favorite thing to do and the source of great distress for my dad! Although my communication skills were excellent when it came to talking to my girlfriends and boyfriends, communication was a bit lacking when trying to explain my teenage thoughts and feelings to my dad. A year later, however, when he became confined to a wheelchair due to multiple sclerosis, somehow we realized the importance of overcoming our communication block and we both searched out ways to restore our communication and in turn our close relationship.

A chronic illness can disrupt communication or it can make a family realize how important it is to everyone's quality of life. When facing difficult situations and life in general, you will benefit from open, honest, considerate means of communication. As my dad and I discovered and this chapter points out, good communication is a skill. Many things will influence your communication style, but if your goal is to improve your circumstances and your relationships, practicing and honing your communication skills will help guarantee that you reach your goal.

Communicating About the Invisible Disease

Fibromyalgia is often referred to as an invisible illness. If something is invisible, other people are not able to use one of their most important communication senses—vision—to help them understand the situation. This is why verbal communication is even more important in the case of fibromyalgia. People with the illness may not have the normal recognizable signs and visual cues to let others know what they are feeling.

Counting on your verbal communication skills to express your feelings is important so that others will understand. If people with fibromyalgia learn how to communicate in a way that connects them to the significant people in their lives, they will ensure that both parties' needs are being met. This will improve the dynamics of your relationships and establish a good system of communication.

Healthy Alternative

Good communication can be a way to help reduce anxiety, minimize anger, and promote positive and supportive interaction. Both speaking and listening are part of good communication. Be sure that what you are saying is …

- Truly what you are feeling.
- Direct and easily understood.
- Worth listening to.
- Respectful of yourself and who you are speaking to.

Because communication takes place on several levels, it is important to understand that *what* you say and *how* you say it are part of the communication process. You communicate your feelings through words *and* gestures. Your family, friends, health-care professionals, and others interpret every aspect of your communication, which influences how they react to you.

For example, if you say, "You need to understand how tired I am today," in a soft, explanatory voice while touching your husband's hand, this communicates that you are requesting his understanding. On the other hand, if you say "You need to understand how tired I am today!" in a frustrated, loud, angry voice, while walking out of the room, the effect is going to be completely different.

In the first example, you are saying that you are tired, but you are also telling your husband that it's not his fault. You are communicating that you would very much appreciate his understanding and that you trust him to accept what you are saying. Then he will know what you are trying to communicate is important. In the second example, the actions speak more loudly than the words. Your husband might interpret your loud, angry voice as "she feels I have done something wrong and that is why she is acting hostile toward me."

By walking away after making that comment, you prevent further communication from taking place and indicate the other person's opinion does not count. When expressing yourself, listen to what you are saying, notice your body language, consider the tone of your voice, and think about whether you are being considerate of the receiver's feelings and needs.

Remember these important elements of communication and evaluate their appropriateness to the situation:

- Body language
- Eye contact
- Voice quality and intonation
- Rhythm and pacing of words
- Sincerity of manner
- Directness
- Response to expressions of emotion
- Self-confidence
- Setting, time, and place
- Sensitivity to others' feelings
- Clarity of message

Honing Your Communication Skills

In today's busy world, communication happens in so many different ways, with so many different people, that it is easy to forget what it takes to be a good communicator. Taking the time to practice open, honest communication, and discussing subjects to prevent miscommunication really important. There are rewards from learning how to practice better communication. Good communication can help with the following:

- Reduce stress and put someone at ease.

- Save time and energy.

- Promote greater understanding of each person's feelings.

- Build closer relationships.

- Remove obstacles.

- Reinforce and clarify feelings about a subject.

- Express concerns and emotional feelings toward someone.

- Give support that can result in therapeutic outcomes.

- Help to educate.

- Inspire and create hope.

- Express beliefs that are paramount to who you are.

- Encourage further communication.

- Get feedback to ensure correct understanding.

As you will learn throughout this chapter, although it might take some time to become a good communicator, if you practice it until it becomes natural, the benefits will definitely outweigh the initial challenges.

Talking About Fibromyalgia

Good communication is a solution to many of the issues and situations that you and your family will face after a fibromyalgia diagnosis. It is often during these difficult times that communication becomes challenging. If you can recognize communication obstacles and apply new communication skills and patterns, you will improve your chances of effective communication. Be aware of the communication obstacles discussed in the following sections.

Different Communication Styles

Communication styles differ greatly depending on your personality, your environment, and even your mood. Christopher L. Heffner, M.S., of Southern Illinois University, suggests that everyone can display different styles of communication depending on a variety of circumstances. However, most people fall into one of three main communication styles: passive, assertive, or aggressive.

Recognizing the style that most resembles your communication technique will help you better understand how others perceive you through interactions.

♦ **Passive.** Passive communicators put the feelings of others before themselves, often being apologetic and avoiding eye contact.

♦ **Assertive.** Assertive communicators stand up for themselves while maintaining respect for others. They speak in a firm voice and maintain eye contact.

♦ **Aggressive.** Aggressive communicators stand up for their rights, but they are not concerned if they violate the rights of others. They often speak in a loud voice with uptight mannerisms.

Different communication styles can be indicative of gender differences. Men often speak in terms of things and attempt to give information, whereas women talk about people and relate best to expressing feelings and emotions. If a man is not able to express his emotions, you can ask him to describe how he is feeling in other ways. He might be better at communicating his feelings through his actions. Let him know that his feelings are very important to you and help him (by listening and being very understanding) to express what he is feeling. If the woman is reacting to things in overly emotional terms, the man can point out the basic realities of the situation and try to deal with them less emotionally. Emotions must be expressed, but be careful when certain emotions start to cloud the facts.

> **Healthy Alternative**
>
> If your emotions become overwhelming and you feel unable to express yourself rationally and coherently, take time to cool off. Write your thoughts and feelings down in a notebook and reflect upon how these feelings should be expressed so that you can gain the support of others, instead of putting them off.

Other relationships have innate tendencies for bias communication. For example, in a parent/child relationship, the parent speaks from a position of power and is often assertive when communicating with their child. However, when a child becomes an adult, a shift in the relationship occurs and it is appropriate for the child's communication style to change. If the parent becomes ill and the child assumes the role of caregiver, parent and child must openly discuss what this new relationship means. The style of communication used will influence whether or not good communication will take place and if the parties involved will be able to adjust.

When an individual becomes ill, it is not unusual to feel dependent on someone else. In these circumstances it is easy to assume a passive communication style. If you are not able to express your feelings and ideas in an open but assertive way, not only will your communication deteriorate, but so will your relationship. Whether you are sick or not, meaningful communication will only happen when both parties are practicing assertive communication with compassion and trust.

Not Asking for Help

Those with a chronic illness are often not comfortable admitting their situation or asking for help. If you are in this situation and you know that explaining your experience will help everyone better understand your actions and feelings, don't be afraid to speak up. Make sure that you are being honest and that those around you know that you are not just complaining, but rather trying to keep everyone apprised of your situation. If you ask for help and are appreciative, you can avoid resentment and frustration.

The Symptoms Themselves

Some symptoms of fibromyalgia might make you less capable of or interested in communication. For example, pain or exhaustion may intensify your desire to pull away from others and to bottle up your fears and frustrations inside. If communication is breaking down between you and the members of your family, question whether or not it is caused by cognitive difficulties, depression, anxiety, or your pain.

If any of your symptoms cause you to avoid situations of communication, talk to your health-care professional immediately. To improve your health, you need to have communication and social interaction with others. The more isolated you become, the worse you will feel and the more you will focus on the negative side of things. Interactions with others helps take your mind off your symptoms, allows you to experience things that will lift your mood, and helps you see things from a different perspective. Talking things out will help relieve tensions and help make things clearer.

Healthy Alternative
I have always loved sending and receiving cards. When I first got sick, I received a lot of cards, which let me know that my friends and family were thinking about me. As time went on, the cards stopped. One day I went to the store and bought a bunch of cards—happy birthday, friendship, thank you, funny, sentimental, and even the blank ones with great pictures on the front. I started sending out the cards to people who I didn't get to see as often as I would like. Before I knew it I was getting cards back, and it became a great way to keep in touch and to express feelings that might not have been shared.

Physical Separation

Actual physical separation can affect communication. If there are reasons for you to be apart from your family and friends, communication might cease.

If fibromyalgia has made you less mobile and unable to see friends, or you spend great amounts of time in your room away from your family, be aware of challenges that may come about. Schedule time to be together or find new ways to keep in touch. Talk about things that don't always revolve around your illness. Be sure that the conversation covers everyone's interests. Even if you aren't feeling good, spending time talking with friends and loved ones can be a very important aspect of improving your health and outlook.

Healthy Alternative
When I was spending a great deal of time at home, my husband would occasionally come into our room and announce that it was time to take a joyride. He would bring me my disguise, including a baseball cap, a pair of sunglasses, and a coat, and we would get into the car and just drive. It didn't matter where we went, it got me out of the house and gave us the opportunity to talk about anything other than my fibromyalgia!

Less Than Truthful

Not expressing yourself truthfully or not using direct vocabulary can cause misunderstandings. When it comes to your health, you need to be honest with yourself and everyone else. Do not push yourself beyond your capabilities, but do not stop trying to do things. Make an effort when you can, but take care of yourself when your body is communicating its need to rest. When something of importance is expressed, it is often helpful if you repeat it a second time so that there is less opportunity for misinterpretation.

Fast Fact _____

Use a pregnant pause (a moment of silence), for two communication effects. The first is when you want to collect your thoughts and give the person you are speaking to a moment to digest what you are saying. The second is after a discussion has come to a decision point and you want to force the other person into speaking their thoughts before you speak yours.

Misplaced Fear or Aggression

Misplaced fear or aggression can be interpreted by your family in ways that will discourage communication. You will weather the difficult times of this illness better if you are not ashamed to express your fears and anxieties. It is important to eagerly look for ways to explore solutions, to discuss your options with others, and to ask for help. Do not keep your feelings bottled up inside. There are times when you will need to vent or even cry. Let the members of your family know that it is helpful if they sometimes just listen.

Be sure that your family interprets your comments correctly. Ask them to repeat what they hear you say. If it is not correct, you will have another opportunity to better explain yourself. If you experience negative emotions, confide your feelings and worries to a person who is likely to understand and whom you can trust. If you feel uncomfortable talking about certain subjects with a family member or friend, you might need to reach out to a more formal helper—clergy, family health-care professional, social worker, counselor, or psychologist.

One-Way Communication

Communication cannot go in just one direction. The feelings and needs of all parties must be addressed and met. Along with communicating these feelings, you must also discuss ways to improve the situation. It is much more constructive to not only point out the problems, but to come up with ways to eliminate them. Be sure you are expressing your feelings in a way that you do not make the people around you feel like you are blaming them for the feelings you have.

Remember, even though you need the support and understanding of your family and friends, they also need _you_ to see things from their perspective. Put yourself in their position and understand how they must be feeling. Even if you are dealing with a chronic illness, don't be discouraged. You are still able to help meet the needs of those around you. Don't forget to listen to what others are saying to you.

Nonassertive Behavior

Your communication style can change in the face of a chronic illness. A loss of self-esteem and a sense of hopelessness can make you unknowingly present poor body language, gestures, and facial expressions that communicate anguish and a sense of losing control. These actions, whether they are intentional or not, might make others uncomfortable and unwilling to be around you. If you choose to use negative words, everything around you becomes more negative. Pain can cause you to physically become hunched over and draw your body inward, expressing your discomfort and communicating to others a desire to be left alone.

Don't ignore your pain, but try to recognize what effect it can have on your communication. Try using more positive words than negative ones and practice expressing open body language. "Negative speak" can result in "negative behavior."

Picture This/Lessons Learned

Picture This:

When I first became ill with fibromyalgia, I believed my husband had no idea what it felt like to suffer with constant pain. I used to wish that he could just feel what it was like for a few minutes so that I would know that he didn't think I was making this up or that I was exaggerating.

One day I overheard him talking to a friend and he said, "… when *we* got fibromyalgia, things changed. You can't imagine what it is like to be in constant pain."

I then realized that our communication had been so comprehensive that not only did my husband understand what I was feeling, but he was feeling it right along with me.

Lesson Learned:

Communication can take the place of actually experiencing something to understand it.

Expressing Your Feelings

Expressing your feelings is one part of communication. But not only do you need to express yourself, you also need to decide with whom you will share these feelings and thoughts. It is important to pick a good listener if you feel like you just need to talk. You need to discuss solution options with someone who is willing to help you identify opportunities. Sometimes there is one person you feel most comfortable confiding in. But don't assume that it has to be just one person. Different people in your life may play different roles, at different times, in helping you deal with the need to express yourself.

There are times when you need someone who will constantly remind you of all the hope there is for a better future; at other times, you will need help to find the source of a problem. Do not waste your time talking to someone who is always negative or refuses to listen to what you are saying. If such a person exists in your immediate family, you (and/or your family) might have to seek professional help with your communication problems to come to terms with ways to promote mutual understanding.

Fast Fact _____

When you communicate with others, your words influence feelings, behaviors, thoughts, and even biochemistry. Humor can increase communication and can be a nonthreatening way of getting others to listen to you and to allow you to express a particular thought or feeling in a relaxed way.

One of the hardest parts about dealing with a chronic illness can be telling your friends and peers. Not knowing how people might react to your news can be a bit concerning. Uncertainty is part of life (health condition or not), and you need to accept that some things are beyond your control. It is better to confront the issue and explain things to people yourself. Their reaction has nothing to do with you, but rather with their own abilities to deal with health issues. How they perceive the situation will affect them. Your true friends will be there to give you support and acceptance.

Another great way to express yourself is through humor. If you can laugh at something that might otherwise seem negative, the humor can make the situation more palatable! Several years ago, I used to share "fibro funnies" with other fibromyalgia patients over the Internet. Some of the humor was only funny to us because we could relate to these odd experiences and attacks of fibro fog, so the group could commiserate and laugh together! One of my favorites was about a woman and her husband who were driving home one day and the car in front of them pulled out in front of another car. When the second car slowed up to avoid the bad driver, the first car honked its horn. The woman commented to her husband, "Can you believe it, that car barked at them!" I could relate to her because I have actually put the milk in the cupboard and the cookies in the refrigerator!

Following is a test you can take to evaluate how comfortable you are talking about fibromyalgia. For each question, circle the answer that you feel applies to you.

Expressing Your Feelings

The people who know that I have fibromyalgia are …

1. No one

2. Just my immediate family

3. My friends

4. My family and friends

5. Everyone who knows me

6. Everyone, even strangers

If I am seeking advice, I will go to …

1. No one

2. Just my immediate family

3. Just my friends

4. My family and friends

5. Everyone who knows me

6. Everyone, even strangers

If I need help, I will go to …

1. No one

2. Just my immediate family

3. Just my close friends

4. My family and friends

5. Everyone who knows me

6. Everyone, even strangers

If I am feeling down, I will …

1. Avoid everyone

2. Turn to my family

3. Turn to my friends

4. Turn to a professional

5. Turn to someone at work

6. Turn to someone who does not know me well

If while talking I started to cry, I would feel …

1. Humiliated and embarrassed

2. Silly

3. Comfortable that it was okay, but I would try to stop quickly

4. Comfortable that it was okay to cry, and I would not feel guilty

5. Relieved that I could express my feelings and continue crying and sobbing until I felt completely better

6. Sobbing uncontrollably and feeling the need to explain why I was reacting in such a way to anyone who is around

If you selected mostly statements marked with smaller numbers (1 or 2), you may not be very open and forthright with your feelings. You might be keeping things bottled up inside, avoiding opportunities to create lines of communication.

If you selected more of the middle numbers (3, 4, or 5), you are probably fairly open with others and recognize that your feelings and illness are nothing to be ashamed of. Family and friends can play a huge role in helping us deal with a chronic illness. You are open to communication, but you realize that there are times when it is not appropriate to share everything with everyone.

If you often selected answer number 6, you might be overcompensating and looking for compassion and acceptance from anyone who will give it. Your openness might have gone beyond what is appropriate. You might not have developed good communication with your family and friends, and so you are trying to find someone who is willing to listen.

What If We Just Don't Agree?

There will be times that you just don't agree with the people in your life. This doesn't have to be a bad thing if you can communicate through your disagreement. But how do you know if you are fighting effectively? Here are some tips:

◆ If the issue is trivial, it might not be worth an argument.

◆ Pick a good time. Don't fight right before you go to bed or when one of you is on their way out of the house.

◆ Make sure you are both fighting about the same thing.

◆ Be direct and concise with your statements. (Never use the silent treatment!)

- Stay on the subject and stay in the present. (Don't bring up things that made you angry days, weeks, or months ago.)

- Don't use accusations or bring up areas of personal sensitivity.

- Be understanding and open to the other's perspective.

- If you can see a way to compromise, suggest it!

- Don't be afraid to admit when you are wrong.

- Come to a resolution that is either a temporary or permanent solution.

- Stick to whatever is agreed on.

- Kiss and make up. (Or whatever is appropriate!)

What Do I Need to Tell My Family?

One of the most important aspects of improving your health is to have good communication with your family. Because illness can affect many aspects of your life, it is obvious that it will also affect the members of your family. You must understand that you did not choose to have this illness come into your family's life, and there is no benefit in placing blame on yourself or anyone else. It is important to focus your concentration on ways to help everyone in the family adapt to this new situation, to learn from it, and to allow it to open up new opportunities that would not have been recognizable or even possible without having to face this kind of challenge. Look on the positive side of things and focus on working together as a family unit that can identify problems, develop and implement plans, and successfully achieve solutions.

When an illness disrupts the way a family operates, it is imperative that everyone works together to redefine roles, to establish a new family order, and to outline expectations and responsibilities. A family conference or weekly discussion can help eliminate resentment, help establish a structure for getting things done, and allow each person a specific time to share information and feelings. Establishing a venue for communication assures everyone in the family an opportunity to express themselves and to have the entire family involved in resolving conflicts.

One of the main challenges that a family has to face when one of its members becomes ill with fibromyalgia is how to redivide tasks. People with fibromyalgia may no longer be able to do some of the things that were once just normal activities. It is okay to switch certain responsibilities with someone else in the family. Roles that may have been divided by gender may now be divided by the "ability to provide."

Certain limitations caused by fibromyalgia are temporary. If you take a break from the activities that are making your symptoms worse, in time you will start taking part in them again. If your family needs extra help, often friends, church members, and others will volunteer. And don't underestimate the abilities of children; it is important that young children know how they fit in and what they can do to be helpful.

Picture This/Lessons Learned

Picture This:

It can be helpful to find unique and personal ways to communicate your feelings. For example: "I feel like I have been run over by [1 to 100] trucks." If you tell your family that today it feels like 10 trucks, they will know that you are doing better than the day before when you expressed your pain level as being hit by 75 trucks!

Lessons Learned:

Coming up with unique and personal ways to help communicate to your family can add humor, make yourself better understood, help your family to better relate to *how* you are feeling, make your communication more personal, and give you a more specific way to express yourself than just saying, "I feel bad today."

The Family Discussion

It is a good idea to establish specific times when the family can sit down together. You will want to discuss ways that each person can contribute and ways to adapt to the new dynamics in the family's relationships. There are several things that will make the family discussions more successful and help to make family communication better:

◆ Everyone needs to promise to be honest. Hiding or lying about facts to protect each other only leads to misunderstanding. Be sure that you are communicating directly and openly to all family members.

◆ Everyone in the family needs to be a part of the communication process. This includes children, the main caregiver, and you. By sharing information, each member of the family will have a stronger sense of purpose and understanding.

◆ Do not underestimate how much people enjoy being helpful. Most people like to contribute, so do not be ashamed to ask for help and accept it with gratitude.

◆ You need to find a way to accurately communicate how your fibromyalgia is affecting you and how you are feeling at any particular time. By letting your family know exactly how you are feeling, you will let them know what they can expect from you at that particular moment.

There are many things you can do to help ensure that your family is understanding, supportive, accepting, and active in helping you improve your health. The following are some ideas for you to think about:

◆ Help your family become knowledgeable about the medical aspects of fibromyalgia: what it is, how it is diagnosed, what the symptoms are, and how the person with fibromyalgia is affected.

One way to accomplish this is to have someone accompany you to your doctor appointments. Ask your health-care professional to explain the illness and help your family member understand that this illness is not in your head and that the symptoms are very real. Ask your health-care professional to give your family member written materials that can further explain this illness.

◆ Provide your family with written materials that speak directly to them. Sometimes it is good to start out by just sharing short articles out of a newspaper or a magazine. As they become more interested, you can share books and videos that will help them learn more about and accept what you are living with.

Not all books and videos share the same message. Be sure that you feel comfortable with the information and how it is presented before sharing it with others.

◆ Encourage your family to take steps to deal with the issues and problems that they are facing. Your family might want to seek out professional help. Seeing a counselor, social worker, or member of the clergy can be very helpful.

◆ Be supportive if family members need to seek help for themselves. Everyone has their own needs, and it is healthy to ask for help, especially from someone who is an expert in the area of your concerns.

◆ Ask your family to help you keep your family life as positive as possible. If everyone is working together to focus on the positive and truly help each other believe that things will get better, you greatly increase your chances that this will happen!

◆ Let your family know that you will help out and take as much responsibility as you can. When you are up to it, be sure that you keep this promise.

Everyone appreciates someone who is trying to do her best, despite adversity. By helping when you can, your family will better understand those times when you cannot.

◆ Talk to your family about things other than your health. Be sure that your relationships have more than just one focus. Show an interest in their life.

If you limit the amount of time you spend talking about your health, your family will be more open to talking about it when it is most important. There will be times when the family will need to discuss the things that will help you get better and times when you will need them just to listen. If at other times you can have conversations that expand your relationship, your family will know that when you talk about your health situation, you really need them to be there for you.

Recognizing Your Family's Needs

Everyone has needs that can be met through various avenues of communication. Remember that if the members of your family feel that their needs are being met, they will be much more likely to want to help meet your needs. Keep in mind that everyone …

- ◆ Needs to have others listen to them.

- ◆ Needs an attentive listener.

- ◆ Needs to know that the listener respects what they are telling them.

- ◆ Needs emotional support.

- ◆ Needs an appropriate touch to be a part of communication.

- ◆ Needs to tell others how their actions are affecting them, without blaming or causing hurt.

- ◆ Needs a safe place to express their thoughts, feelings, dreams, and aspirations.

- ◆ Needs communication to help them build self-esteem and create confidence to take on challenges, knowing that others are there backing them.

- ◆ Feels good when someone invites them into a conversation by asking them a question.

- ◆ Needs reassurance that they are loved and that a support system exists for them.

- ◆ Benefits by talking to others who know what they are going through.

- ◆ Benefits from laughing and having fun.

- ◆ Needs to be accepted for who they are.

A family can be a safe place to express your thoughts, feelings, dreams, and aspirations, as long as open, safe communication exists. By evaluating who in your family is having their communication needs met, you and your family will recognize where good communication is taking place and also identify problems and ways to correct those issues. If there is disagreement about a certain person's needs being met, this is a perfect opportunity to discuss the situation openly and honestly and to come to a resolution.

Family Members (Including Yourself)						
Others in my family listen to me.						
I have at least one attentive listener.						
The listener respects what I am telling him or her.						
I receive emotional support.						
I receive appropriate touch.						
I am able to tell others how their actions are affecting me without blaming or causing hurt.						
I have a safe place to express my thoughts, feelings, dreams, and aspirations.						
I experience communication that builds self-esteem and creates confidence to take on challenges.						
Others invite me into conversations by asking me questions.						
I get reassurance that I am loved.						
I have the opportunity to talk to others who know what I am going through.						
I laugh and have fun.						
I feel I am accepted for the person I am.						

To evaluate your family's communication, take the test in Appendix C.

The Least You Need to Know

◆ Good communication can be a way to help reduce anxiety, minimize anger, and promote positive and supportive interactions.

◆ Good communication is a solution to many of the issues and situations that you and your family will face after a fibromyalgia diagnosis.

◆ When an illness disrupts the way a family operates, it is imperative that everyone works together to redefine roles, to help establish a new family order, and to outline expectations and responsibilities.

Chapter 6

Creating a Family Communication Plan

In This Chapter

◆ Creating a Family Communication Plan

◆ Knowing the correct questions to address in the plan

◆ Commenting about communication by health-care professionals

◆ Communicating with yourself

In the previous chapter, you learned the importance of good communication. You identified what specific areas of communication you need to improve and what areas are working well. The next step is to create a Family Communication Plan that addresses the needs of your family as a whole. By identifying tasks and determining who is best suited to execute them, there will be no confusion about who is going to do what. Discussions about the difficulty or amount of time a certain task takes can also help ensure that your family members all feel the plan is fair and that they can accomplish their responsibilities. Major family decisions can also be addressed in the development of a communication plan.

It's Great When a Plan Comes Together

First, you need to become familiar with the things you can do to ensure that the communication plan goes smoothly. It is imperative that every family member is included in the discussions. It is to the whole family's advantage if everyone is encouraged to participate, so no one feels left out. Even small children can help by becoming active participants in the discussions and activities.

The development of a Family Communication Plan will take time. Schedule discussions at convenient times for everyone in the family. When you hold a family discussion, one person should be responsible for taking notes so ideas can be written down and referred to at a later date. It might be necessary to include a mediator (such as a social worker or other person outside of the family) to help negotiate the family through sensitive issues.

Picture This/Lessons Learned

Picture This:

When I was first diagnosed with fibromyalgia and I realized that I was going to have to stop working for a while, I had terrible fears of what the financial repercussions were going to be. We had always been a two-income family and I knew that major adjustments would need to be made. My husband and I decided to have several discussions where we wrote down all the unnecessary expenditures we could think of and together developed a financial budget that fit our new circumstances.

Lessons Learned:

By creating a plan, we were able to easily adjust to having only one income. Many of the expenses that go along with a job were also eliminated (extra gasoline, work clothes, and lunches out), so my fears of poverty were relieved and I was able to take the time I needed to rest and work on my health.

No matter what, each person must be committed to listening carefully and with an open mind to what everyone has to say. There is usually more than one way to solve a problem. It is important that everyone be willing to work toward a compromise. Make sure that new ideas are explored at each meeting and that all the facts are presented and evaluated before a final decision is made.

Issues that need to be addressed when someone in the family is dealing with a chronic illness can leave other members of the family angry, confused, and isolated. If tempers are raised, be sure to take a break so that everyone can calm down before he or she says something they might regret later. At the end of each meeting, review what was decided and what is being left to be decided at future meetings.

Creating the Plan

As a family group, address each of the following questions and write down the thoughts of every participant. After all the questions have been answered, go back to each question and come to a family agreement as to how that situation should be dealt with. If your family is limited to three or fewer people, you might want to include friends, professionals, and any others who are willing to help in your discussion. Remember, everyone should be considered equal participants in the plan. It's also important to make sure that *you* are involved in the implementation of the plan.

Questions to ask:

- What tasks (household chores, errands, meal preparation, and so on) need to get done that aren't getting done?

- Who is the most capable person to perform each task?

- How long should a certain task be assigned before a new family member takes over that task? Keep track of these decisions on a calendar or chart.

- Who can act as the primary caregiver?

- What are the main responsibilities of the primary caregiver?

- Is the caregiver able to physically perform the necessary care? Be sure that the main caregiver is not putting his or her health at risk.

- What special arrangements (time to go to water therapy, quiet time when you are in pain, time to go to a support group meeting, and so on) need to be made so that you have time to focus on your health?

- What needs to be changed to make sure the family's needs are being addressed? Make sure that there are still plenty of positive, fun things that bring the family together.

- What efforts are being made so each child feels he or she is getting the attention they need?

- What financial issues need to be addressed? Is there a need to make career changes or reevaluate spending priorities?

- Is there a need to find additional help (housekeeper, babysitter, dog walker, gardener, and so on)?

- Is there a need to make major changes (move to a different size/type of home, have other family members move in to help, change previously made plans, and so on) in your family's lifestyle?

- What are the special needs of each family member that should be protected? If a member has a special talent or love for a particular hobby, the family should try to work out ways that this person can continue with this activity.

- Is there someone who can ensure that the family remains positive and happy? Many families have a person who is known for being the cheerleader. This person could be very helpful in keeping the family's spirits up.

- What special abilities (such as health-care professionals, tutor, financial advisor, member of the clergy) will need to be available to the family?

- Where can you find people with these abilities?

- What will your family's future be like? Set reasonable goals that give everyone something to look forward to. Plan special family rewards for achieving or maintaining certain family needs.

Making Commitments

Every family has disagreements, but a family committed to practicing open, honest, and ongoing communication will find that this practice can reduce misunderstandings and resentment. Effective communication will benefit every member of the family.

One way to ensure effective communication is for everyone in the family to *agree* to be a part of the Family Communication Commitment Pact.

By agreeing to participate in the family pact, each family member agrees to work toward utilizing good communication skills. Because it takes time to develop good communication skills, everyone must pledge to put in the necessary effort and time to become well versed in these skills.

Pain Signal

People interpret what they hear based on their own experiences. If you are experiencing negative reactions to what someone is saying, ask yourself if you actually understand what he or she is saying. Often we are hurt by what someone has said without understanding what the person is actually trying to communicate to us. Don't be afraid to clarify a point if you are confused by what someone else is saying. Often it is miscommunication that is the real problem.

Family Communication Commitment Pact

Prior to signing the Commitment Pact, be sure that everyone understands each aspect of the agreement and that he or she is freely committing to uphold the statements of the pact.

As a member of the _____ family, I promise to make every effort to practice good communication skills, which include the following:

♦ Listening intently and actively to the other members of my family. Listening promotes more meaningful and satisfying conversations. Although I am listening, I will make sure that I am receiving the communicator's underlying message.

♦ Recognizing that everyone is entitled to have and express his or her own feelings. I will not trivialize anyone's opinions or feelings.

♦ When a family member asks to talk to me, I will give her my undivided attention as soon as I can.

♦ Scheduling time for serious discussions in a place that is quiet and private, at a time that is convenient for everyone involved.

♦ Apologizing without hesitation if I am sorry for something I said or did.

♦ Not responding to comments by other family members with anger or sarcasm. I will not preach, nag, or pretend that I "know exactly how they feel."

♦ Avoiding negative, emotional comments such as "You are wrong" or "That's a dumb idea!"

♦ Negotiating and compromising in all conversations. I will learn to come to agreement on issues without getting emotional.

♦ Keeping my language and sentence structure simple and easy to understand.

♦ Helping to ensure that my message is being understood, and its importance is recognized, by repeating the key messages several times.

♦ Making sure that I am communicating in both directions—as the speaker and as the listener.

Signatures: Date: _____

_____

_____

_____

Our society gives great credence to the written word. If something is in writing, it holds much more weight than a simple verbal statement. People are much more likely to keep a promise that has been written down than one which has been verbally exchanged! At first it may seem odd that a "family" would need to put a promise to one another in writing, but every group of people, whether it is a family or a corporation, benefits by establishing guidelines and structure for the way it functions.

Building family communication is one of the most important activities you can do to help improve your quality of life. If your family is willing to address difficult situations and decisions and take the time to work together to assure that everyone is able to voice his or her opinions and play a role in the family's activities, a more harmonious environment will result and everyone will benefit.

Picture This/Lessons Learned

Picture This:

Sandy's brother Fred could not understand why his sister was now unable to take care of all the family responsibilities she eagerly managed before she became sick with fibromyalgia. No amount of talking seemed to bridge the gap that was growing wider between them. Finally, the problem became so bad that they stopped talking completely. Weeks went by and then months and then years and the two remained estranged. Just by chance, one day Fred was standing in line at a market where he picked up a magazine containing an article explaining the symptoms of fibromyalgia. Although his sister had not been able to help him understand her illness, seeing it in print gave the words authority and helped him better understand what it is like to live with the illness. Fred called his sister and they agreed to get together to talk. Although they still have gaps in their communication, that article brought them back together and gave them a second chance at working things out.

Lessons Learned:

Never underestimate the "authority" of the written word. If you are having trouble helping your family understand what you are feeling and experiencing, it can be helpful to provide them with written information, especially materials that are compiled by an authority. (Remember though, you can lead a horse to water but you can't make it drink!)

Additional Tips to Promote Good Family Communication

Here are some practical tips that are guaranteed to improve communication between members of your family:

- Humor is an excellent way to disarm angry, cruel words. "When you say that, you sound just like Tom Cruise!"

- Expressing thoughts that you usually only think. "I have something to tell you, but I am afraid of how you are going to react."

- Affirming what the person is saying when he or she is pointing out your faults. "You are right; I am a big jerk, but let me try to make it up to you."

- Pointing out areas that you *do* agree on when you are discussing things that you don't agree on. "I am not sure if I can agree with you on that point, but I do agree that we both are working very hard to support this family."

- Don't always give your opinion; ask and listen for family members' thoughts. "Can you give me an example of what you would like to see happen?"

- Stop using words that are upsetting to a family member. "I won't call you a child anymore; I will recognize that you are now a teenager."

What Health-Care Professionals Say

When we are looking for answers to our questions or information on certain topics, we turn to experts for their opinion. Here's what some of the foremost fibromyalgia health-care professionals say about communication:

> "There is a tendency to shut out the family and caring ones because of your pain. Essentially you shut out the world because of your pain. Instead of the pain being less, the pain is actually noticed more because the world around you has shrunk so small that there is nothing else in it except you and your pain.

> "Don't shut out your relationships. Keep them in your world. Let your family help you and allow yourself to play an active role in educating and communicating with your family."

—Mark J. Pellegrino, M.D., Physical Medicine and Rehabilitation

> "The practitioner should schedule a prolonged visit or a series of visits when they are first seeing a person with fibromyalgia or they suspect a diagnosis of fibromyalgia. The time invested in the beginning of the health-care professional–patient relationship pays tremendous long-term dividends for the practitioner and the patient. It is necessary to spend this time in order for the health-care professional to understand precisely what is bothering the patient and for the patient to

understand the goals of (and rationale for) treatment. During these visits, it is important to explore the symptoms that the individual is experiencing, the impact of the disorder on the patient's life, the patient's perception of what is causing these symptoms, and the stressors that may be exacerbating the illness.

"Once these goals have been accomplished, the patient should be educated about the nondestructive nature of this condition, as well as the fact that meaningful improvement rarely occurs without active participation on the patient's part— the patient must know that there is no 'magic bullet' for treatment."

—Daniel Clauw, M.D., University of Michigan

"One of the most important things a physician can do is to greet a patient with a smile, communicating to them that there are ways to manage fibromyalgia. A person with fibromyalgia will have an increased chance of improvement if their physician helps to restore their self-confidence and helps provide them with motivation and hope. Open communication between a patient and their physician will promote healthy teamwork."

—Muhammad B. Yunus, M.D., University of Illinois, Peoria

"One of the most powerful communication devices is empathy. If you can come to understand how your spouse is feeling you will be able to improve your communication. Try developing a system which allows your spouse to express the level of pain she is feeling. You could use a 1 to 100 rating scale, which will give her chance to really pinpoint the level of pain she is experiencing."

—Robert Williams, M.D., Arthritis Consultants

Experts agree that fibromyalgia can place a lot of strain on relationships between a patient and the ones caring for him or her. According to one study, most of the personal needs of the patient are fulfilled by just one or two people—often a spouse or a physician. When communication breaks down, the person with fibromyalgia becomes more and more isolated and less likely to receive the support necessary to get better.

Don't Forget to Communicate with Yourself!

To effectively communicate with others, you first need to "communicate" with yourself. Reflecting on your own feelings, experiences, and goals will help you to evaluate what steps you want to take in the future and prepare you to voice an opinion about the direction you want to take.

There is no one "right" way to communicate with yourself. There are times when you will want to review facts in your mind or write them down to help you make a decision, and other times when you will want to try to clear your mind, sit quietly, and see where your subconscious takes you. There are many ways you can talk to yourself. You can …

♦ Keep an activities journal.

♦ Write a letter to yourself.

♦ Compose a poem.

♦ Make lists of accomplishments and positive thoughts.

♦ Write a story about your dreams.

♦ Recognize your mistakes and figure out ways to avoid making the same mistakes in the future.

> **Healthy Alternative**
>
> Communication comes in many different forms. The lyrics of a song are a type of communication. When you are feeling down, listen to music that has lyrics that can make you happy. If you want to relax, listen to song that has a message of calm and serenity.

♦ Find your "personal supporter" or your self-esteem and listen to what it says.

♦ Talk to yourself as you would like others to talk to you.

♦ Put yourself in someone else's shoes and pretend to be that person, so you can better understand his feelings.

♦ Practice saying things that you want to express to others, so that when the time comes you will be ready to say what you are feeling. (This should include saying no.)

♦ Be kind to yourself and verbally let yourself off the hook when you are being too hard on yourself.

♦ Meditate.

♦ Visualize how you would like things to be and write down your thoughts.

♦ Repeat positive thoughts over and over to yourself.

♦ If a thought comes to you and you are afraid that you will not remember it, stop and write it down.

By communicating with yourself, you can begin to take control of your thoughts and focus on the positive direction you want your life to take.

The Least You Need to Know

◆ Everyone in the family needs to participate in creating the Family Communication Plan.

◆ Openly discuss questions that can identify problems, tasks, and goals and come to a family decision as to how these issues are going to be addressed.

◆ A family committed to practicing open, honest, ongoing communication will find that this practice can reduce misunderstandings and resentment. Effective communication benefits every member of the family.

◆ Remember to talk to yourself as you would like others to talk to you.

Chapter 7

Preparing for Your Doctor's Appointment

In This Chapter

- Becoming a savvy patient
- Preparing your symptom history
- Preparing questions for your doctor's appointment
- Relying on memory is not enough—take notes!
- Learning what to expect from your doctor
- Recognizing the importance of an advocate

One of the most important members of your health-care team is your primary care physician. It is to your benefit to find a doctor with whom you feel you can create a mutually beneficial relationship. A health-care professional's job is to provide you with medical advice, treatment, and hope. Your job is to help the health-care provider help you. This is not an adversarial or one-sided relationship. You cannot expect your doctor to wave a magic wand and make you better. You will benefit most if you understand the tools as well as the limitations that affect your physician's ability to treat you.

Over the past 10 to 20 years, the medical community's knowledge about fibromyalgia has increased greatly. Today, it is easier to find a health-care professional who is knowledgeable and interested in treating a person with fibromyalgia. After you have found that person, you must fulfill your role—and practice being a good patient.

To get the medical help you need, you must be a savvy patient. This includes knowing how to find a good doctor, being well prepared for your appointments, presenting your concerns in an organized and concise manner, and being able to recruit an advocate who can help you with this entire process. You learned how to find a good doctor in Chapter 4; as you move through this chapter, you learn how to be prepared, communicate your concerns, and utilize the help of an advocate. This may all seem overwhelming when you are in desperate need of medical answers and help, but if you learn how to maneuver through the system, the benefits will outweigh the challenges.

Communicating with Your Doctor

Prior to your first doctor's appointment, take the time to write or type your questions and symptoms in an organized format. I suggest you compile two lists—one with information about the symptoms you are experiencing and one with questions you have for your doctor. This is a process that requires concentration. You may want to ask a family member, friend, social worker, community volunteer, or paid assistant to help you with this process.

For your first doctor's visit, be sure to schedule enough time to cover your major concerns. Remember that under most circumstances, a doctor has only enough time to address two or three issues per appointment. Because people with fibromyalgia have multiple symptoms, it is important to prioritize the items on your lists so that you can cover the most important issues during the time your doctor has available. You may also need to make a series of appointments so you can adequately cover each issue. If you aren't sure how to prioritize your concerns, ask your physician to review your list of symptoms and address the most medically important symptoms first.

If you are respectful of your physician's time, you can often ask whether he or she is available to communicate via emergency appointments, telephone, e-mail, office staff, or clinic group meetings. If your current physician is not available to address your needs, you need to find one who is.

When you are at the doctor's office, make sure that you take notes, ask the doctor to write things down for you, or have an advocate (friend or family member) there as a note taker and an extra pair of ears. Oftentimes you will forget or misunderstand what has been said, especially during a rushed appointment. Fibro fog can make your appointment seem like a blur, so if you haven't made arrangements for someone else to record the meeting, you may go home feeling unsure of your physician's suggestions and instructions. Another option is for you to ask the doctor for permission to record the appointment.

Fast Fact _____

Part of being a good patient means you must recognize the boundaries that are inherent to a doctor's appointment:

There are limits on the amount of time the physician can spend with you.

If you present too many problems at once, the physician will not be effective in addressing any of your symptoms or questions.

An understanding physician is important, but you should rely on others to provide you with sympathy and let your physician provide you with medical advice.

Your physician is not psychic! You must communicate your concerns and needs in a direct manner.

Do not ever feel afraid to ask questions and to be open and direct with your physician. Explain to the doctor how you are feeling physically. Give him or her specific examples of your symptoms, how long they have been bothering you, and their level of intensity. Share your emotional state with your physician, too. Your doctor will be better able to treat you if you are honest about feeling depressed, afraid, frustrated, or alone. Your physician needs to know what kind of treatments you have tried in the past and what kinds of treatments you are most comfortable with. If you prefer a more conservative approach to prescription medications, let your physician know that at the outset. Again, your most important task is to create a partnership with your physician—and good open communication is the best way to create that partnership.

Preparing Your Symptom History

In order for your doctor to determine a diagnosis and formulate a treatment plan, he or she will take your complete medical history, listen to your symptom description, and perform a physical examination. It is extremely important to tell your doctor everything *you* feel is significant at the beginning of your appointment, so your doctor can concentrate on what is found during the exam. In order to prepare for your appointment, there are several things you should do.

Healthy Alternative

When is it appropriate to call the doctor and request an immediate appointment? Chest pains, shortness of breath, fainting, sharp pains that worsen with a deep breath, ongoing fever, sudden or sharp abdominal pain, vomiting blood or the appearance of blood in your urine or stool, coughing up yellow mucous, and dizziness or loss of balance are symptoms that should receive immediate medical attention. Also request an immediate appointment if a new symptom has a sudden onset and seems unlike other fibromyalgia symptoms you have experienced.

Begin by keeping an ongoing list of the symptoms you experience and how they affect your life. You will have an easier time compiling these important facts before each doctor visit. These notes will not only help your doctor understand your case, but they can be included in your medical chart. If you are prepared with this information you will save time and be assured that you can accurately communicate your situation to your doctor.

Next, take the time to prepare the following information prior to your doctor's appointment:

♦ Each medical symptom and its date of onset

♦ How often you experience the symptom

♦ How the symptom is affecting your life

♦ All emotional symptoms you are experiencing, and how long you have been feeling that way

♦ The effects these emotional symptoms are having on your life

♦ Each medication you are allergic to and what kind of reaction you have experienced

♦ If you don't have insurance and are paying for your prescriptions out-of-pocket

♦ Your concerns about any type of treatment your doctor may recommend

Because pain is one of the most common symptoms experienced by someone with fibromyalgia, it is helpful to track your pain and keep your physician informed about any changes in pain that you experience. Don't become consumed with writing down every little pain you have, but take general notes once a day and present these notes to your doctor at your appointment. Include the following in your notes:

◆ The type of pain you are experiencing (aching, stabbing, numbness, tingling, burning, and so on)

◆ The level of pain on a scale of one to 10, with 10 being the worst pain possible

◆ The duration of the pain and where it is located on your body

To help you with this task you can make a copy of the diagram below and then shade the area or areas where you are experiencing pain. Complete a new diagram prior to each doctor's appointment.

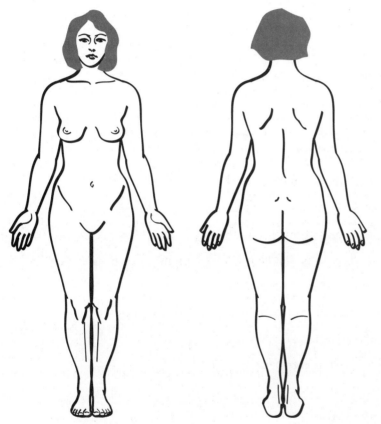

Shade the areas on the figure where you are experiencing pain. Write comments near the shaded areas to help explain the type of pain that you are experiencing.

Additional information that can be of help to your physician includes …

◆ **Past treatments:** drugs, supplements, herbs, physical therapy, acupuncture, exercise, sleep clinics, and so on. Make a note if the treatment was not helpful, somewhat helpful, or very helpful.

◆ **Past physicians:** all physicians you have seen and how long you were under their care. Make a note if you are still seeing other health-care professionals.

Preparing Questions for the Doctor

If you are prepared with well-thought-out questions, you will save time and make the most of your doctor's appointment. Prioritize the following questions and add any questions you have that are not covered here. Remember that it will take more than one appointment before you have all your questions answered.

Priority Questions

What kinds of tests will I have?

What do you expect to find out from these tests?

When will I know the results?

Will my results be mailed to me or should I expect a phone call?

Who will be available to explain the results?

What can cause my condition?

What is my diagnosis?

How will this condition affect me now and in the future?

Should I watch for any particular symptoms and notify you if they occur?

What lifestyle changes should I make?

What are the treatments for my condition?

When will treatment start?

Why has this drug been prescribed?

How do I take it?

Do I take it with or without food?

Can I take it with other medications?

At what time of day should I take it?

How much or how many should I take?

How often should I take it?

What are the short-term side effects?

What are the long-term side effects?

If I experience side effects, what should I do?

How long will I have to take it?

Are there less expensive medications for my condition?

Will this new drug interact with any of the other medicines I am taking?

Are other types of treatments available?

What are the most beneficial treatments?

Should I see other specialists?

What are the risks and side effects associated with treatment?

Are there foods, drugs, or activities I should avoid?

Will my symptoms ever go away completely?

Will I need more tests later?

Where can I go for support?

Where can I go for additional information?

As you add additional questions, keep in mind that it is always appropriate and important to ask your doctor questions about your health. Issues you might find embarrassing are probably nothing new to your doctor. Always ask "How?," "Why?," and "Why not?" The more informed you become, the fewer concerns you will have.

Communicating with Your Doctor

Now that you are well prepared to meet with the doctor, your appointment will be organized and you will be able to clearly express your concerns and expectations. Let your doctor know that you are looking for a partnership, and that you want to work together to achieve positive outcomes. By establishing a long-term, mutually satisfying association, you will receive continuity of care and develop a shared respect for one another.

As you are explaining your health history and symptoms, your doctor needs time to analyze your symptoms and the exam findings, so if he or she appears to be deep in thought, allow some quiet time so you do not interrupt that thinking process.

Remember that sharing information is important, but *listening* is just as important. Always ask the doctor to repeat or clarify information that seems unclear. It is helpful to summarize your understanding of what the doctor has just told you.

If you have researched health-care providers well, you will be meeting with a respected and qualified physician. Although no one knows your body better than you, keep an open mind, follow directions, and let your doctor know if you choose to do something other than what he or she has suggested. Express your willingness to work with the doctor to find a more agreeable treatment, or to change the treatment to better meet your needs. Remember, two heads are better than one!

What You Can Expect from Your Doctor

If you have expectations that your doctor is not able to meet, you will feel disillusioned and let down. Realistic expectations will help you know exactly what you can expect from your doctor. The following is a list of things that your health-care professional can do for you:

- ◆ Your doctor can't guarantee that a particular medication will work for you, but can inform you of the reasons why he or she recommended a specific medication and what may be accomplished by prescribing the drug.

- ◆ Follow-up appointments are designed to determine how you are progressing with specific treatments and to determine what needs immediate attention. For more complex problems, you should schedule a full consultation that will give you more time with the doctor.

- ◆ Your doctor can't guarantee that emergencies won't come up. You may have to reschedule an appointment—but he or she should be able to see you if you have a true emergency.

- ◆ Doctors can't guarantee that your insurance will cover all of your medical needs, but they can be sensitive to the limitations of your insurance policy.

- ◆ Your doctor can't promise always to agree with you or tell you what you want to hear, but does have a responsibility to "first do no harm."

- ◆ Your doctor may not have all the answers, but can refer you to other health-care professionals who can help you with specific problems.

- ◆ You can't expect your doctor to be your friend, but you can expect him or her to treat you with respect and to listen to your concerns and requests.

Making the Most of Your Doctor Visit

After you have met with the doctor, it is important to make use of the advice and help your doctor has offered. If you would like copies of your test results, make arrangements with the doctor's office staff when you check out from your appointment. Once you get home, review your notes, make sure that you understand the directions you have been given, and mark your next appointment on your calendar.

If your doctor wants you to start taking new medications or is refilling your current prescriptions, make sure that you get to the pharmacy right away. If you are taking multiple medications, make sure that you write down which medicines you are to take daily, including how much and when. An inexpensive plastic multi-day pillbox can help you remember when to take your medications. Make notes of any side effects you are experiencing and what type of response you are noticing from the prescribed treatment(s). If you are interested in doing additional research on the medications you are taking, go to www.fda.gov/cder or call 1-888-INFO-FDA.

Keep in mind that even if there is a good reason for changing or stopping a treatment, you can hurt yourself by not following your doctor's directions. If you have concerns about a particular treatment that has been prescribed for you, be honest with your doctor and find out whether there are any negative ramifications if you do not continue that treatment plan. You may need to be weaned off your medications, or you may be able to treat side effects with other treatment options.

Pain Signal

If you are taking prescription medications and notice any adverse reactions, contact your health-care professional immediately. Side effects can include hives, nausea, dizziness, shortness of breath, excessive sleepiness, headache, vomiting, and constipation, to name just a few.

Pain Signal

Everything you put into your body causes a reaction. Everything—food, herbs, vitamins, minerals, or chemical compounds—has an effect on your body. Even a simple food such as shrimp can be lethal to some people. Because everyone reacts differently, it is important that you have as much information as possible to prevent adverse reactions. Don't take chances by "playing doctor" and mixing over-the-counter supplements with prescription drugs without consulting your health-care professional.

Don't forget that even nonprescription treatments (herbs, vitamins, and other supplements) can interact and have adverse reactions with prescription medications. It is better to be safe than sorry—let you doctor know about everything, treatment wise, you are undertaking!

The Role of an Advocate

An advocate can play many roles as a member of your health-care team. Although there are situations where patients are unable to make decisions for themselves and a person can be designated as a *legal* advocate, in this case I am talking about an advocate to help and support you. It is important that this person be someone you trust. An advocate should feel confident and comfortable in helping you with communication, making decisions, and offering physical and emotional support when you need it. Ask your advocate to do research for you and keep you updated on new research findings and treatments.

Your advocate should be someone who is willing to speak up on your behalf and take charge of the situation for short periods of time if you are unable to. Advocates are especially helpful if a patient feels uncomfortable in a situation, because they can step in and act as a mediator, removing the stress of a difficult situation. For example, if your doctor's office staff is not providing the service that your doctor has said they would, your advocate can handle the situation so you will not have to be involved.

One of the most important things an advocate can do for you is to accompany you to a doctor's appointment. It helps to have another person interpret what is said and think of questions to ask.

Before committing to a relationship with someone as an advocate, make sure that you speak in depth to him or her about your wants and needs. Your advocate may have a different perspective than you do, so listen to his or her thoughts about various situations. You do not want an advocate who is negative! The positive attitude and strength of an advocate can help you be positive and strong. Be sure that your advocate is willing to implement your wishes. If you tell your doctor one thing and your advocate tells him something else, your doctor will be confused and you might not end up with the care or treatment you need.

Pain Signal _____

Is your advocate looking out for your best interests? Be aware of the following warning signs:

◆ Your advocate is talking to your doctor behind your back.

◆ Your advocate expresses a different opinion than you discussed together.

◆ You are sure that your doctor said one thing during your appointment and your advocate disagrees with you.

◆ The decisions that you and your doctor have made in the past are not being implemented and you haven't arranged for any changes.

◆ Your advocate is constantly trying to convince you that you are not doing things correctly and that there is a better way to do things.

◆ If your advocate is a family member and you are having disagreements, it is time to find a new advocate!

The Least You Need to Know

◆ One of the most important members of your health-care team is your primary care physician.

◆ Be respectful of the time constraints that exist when visiting a health-care professional. Prioritize your questions, and if necessary, schedule multiple appointments to cover your concerns and needs.

◆ Prior to your doctor's appointment, take the time to write or type your questions and symptom complaints in an organized format.

◆ Keep in mind that even if there is a good reason for changing or stopping a treatment, you can unknowingly hurt yourself by not following your doctor's directions.

◆ An advocate (friend or family member) can accompany you to your doctor's appointment to take notes and listen to what the doctor says.

Chapter 8

Administration

In This Chapter

- ◆ Keeping track of an accurate chart is important
- ◆ Keeping your medical record on file is a good idea
- ◆ Tracking medical tests and procedures
- ◆ Understanding your insurance coverage
- ◆ Changing insurance coverage should be done carefully

Not too long ago my husband was cleaning out the garage when he came upon a large box marked "Sick." When I opened it up, I found an assortment of file folders containing medical records, insurance claim forms, letters, medical bills, and receipts from 1994. It was the administrative remains of my first year with fibromyalgia. As I peered into the box, my heart sank. The memory of my husband and me trying to manage all of that paperwork still haunts me. The fact remains, however, that no matter how sick you are, someone has to take care of the finances and paperwork.

In this chapter, you learn what your administrative responsibilities are and which tasks will be taken care of by the health-care professionals you see. Despite the inconvenience, it is imperative for you or a family member to keep track of your medical bills, to remain updated on your health insurance coverage, and to request copies of your medical records when necessary.

The Medical Chart

The notes that a health-care professional makes while diagnosing and treating his or her patients make up what is known as the medical chart, which is the property of that physician. Patients, however, have a right to access their medical records and a qualified right to amend their records pursuant to the federal privacy regulations of HIPAA (Health Insurance Portability and Accountability Act of 1996).

When you are dealing with an illness, your primary concern is seeking medical assistance to help you feel better, so it is understandable that you might not realize how important your medical record can be to your future. However, it is vital that you keep track of all medical records in your name and know how and when to get copies. Your medical record can have a major impact on your treatment and finances, and can even affect the success of an application for disability. Although health-care professionals take the medical chart very seriously, they are human and can make mistakes, just like anyone else. Those errors can lead to future mistakes regarding your health care. If a physician refers to an incorrect chart, it is possible that he or she will misinterpret your medical situation and even prescribe the wrong treatment.

Fast Fact

Remember, the physician owns the chart and the patient owns the information contained in the chart. That's why the physician needs to maintain possession of the original chart—and why the physician must obtain the patient's authorization to release any information in the chart.

For example, if your chart doesn't have your drug allergies listed correctly, in an emergency situation a decision could be based solely on your *incorrect* chart. If the physician interprets something you say incorrectly and records that misunderstanding, others who review the chart will be referring to incorrect information, too. Let's say you tell your doctor that you are always anxious about your illness. He might note that you reported that you are experiencing anxiety. If what you meant was that your illness causes you concern, your chart will now reflect incorrect information. The only way that something like this can be corrected is if you know what is in your chart and take the appropriate steps to correct any misinformation.

Many individuals have access to your chart and contribute to its contents. This makes it even more likely that a mistake could be made. Problems arise because of poor handwriting, the misinterpretation of a comment, or even a typing mistake during transcription!

Record Access Policies

Realizing the importance of your medical chart is only the beginning. You must also be aware that medical record policies are subject to a patchwork of state and federal laws and regulations. This means that there is no continuity from state to state. For example, nine states do not specify any legal time period that health-care professionals must keep your records, whereas 21 states require retention for 10 years and the remaining states require records be kept between 3 and 7 years.

The American Medical Association has deemed it ethical for a health-care professional to charge a reasonable amount for providing patients with copies of their medical records and tests. Each state has detailed regulations that apply to the health-care professionals in that state. In North Carolina, physicians are allowed to charge 25 cents per page, whereas South Carolina allows 65 cents per page. You need to find out what the laws are in your state.

Although state laws do vary, many states have adopted a general policy similar to the North Carolina Medical Board's "Access to Medical Records" policy. That is, every health-care professional has a duty, on the request of a patient (or the patient's representative), to release a copy of the record in a timely manner to the patient, unless the physician believes that such release would endanger the patient's life or cause harm to another person. This includes medical records received from other physician offices or health-care facilities.

Fast Fact

The American Health Information Management Association (AHIMA) provides a comprehensive listing of each state's policies and how much can be charged, in addition to the statute on which the state law is based (see www.ahima.org).

Most states have provisions that protect an individual's right to confidentiality and to obtain a copy of their medical record. For example, under California law, patients have the right to …

♦ Obtain complete information about their medical condition and care.

♦ Inspect their medical records within five days of making a written request.

♦ Have their medical records kept confidential unless they provide written consent, except in a limited number of circumstances.

♦ Sue any person who unlawfully releases their medical information without written consent.

Copies of your treating physician's policies should be made available to you, in writing, when you first visit that physician. Request a copy, if necessary. Most physicians or health facilities require you to make your request for copies in writing, and many have a specific form, such as an "Authorization for Release of Health-Care Information," that you must accurately complete. Don't be put off by this system; it is in place to protect you, and is a necessary step if you wish to receive a copy of your records.

Recently, some states have begun enacting new laws to ensure that no charges are made if the record is requested for immunization documentation required for school admission, or for the purposes of supporting a claim or appeal under the provision of the Social Security Act or any federal or state needs-based benefit program such as Medical Assistance, Rite Care, Temporary Disability Insurance, and Unemployment Compensation.

Although you can request your records on your own, there are companies that can, for a fee, retrieve your records for you. Many of these companies are able to obtain your medical records within a week's time.

Why You Need Copies

There are many reasons why you might want to access your medical record. It is a history of the management of your health care by each medical professional you have seen. It records what was done (and not done) by a specific health-care provider. The record helps preserve the facts of your diagnosis, treatment, and laboratory and other medical tests, as well as the communication between your doctor and you.

In addition to checking the accuracy, you might need copies of your medical records for the following reasons:

◆ If you are being treated by multiple physicians, it is standard policy that copies of your medical records and medical tests be provided to, and coordinated by, your family physician or main health-care professional. The documents are usually transferred from one caregiver to the other directly. You can, however, request the records and provide them yourself for other health-care professionals. (Remember: when sharing this information, it should remain confidential and you should be sensitive whom you share it with.)

◆ If you are severing ties with a particular physician, you may want to get a copy of your records for reference by future health-care professionals.

◆ If your physician is retiring or selling his or her practice, the new doctor is required to continue maintaining the records. However, you may want to request a copy of the records, so that you know they will be available to you in the future.

◆ If your attorney or other representative needs your medical records for litigation, he or she may ask you to either sign a request-for-copies form or to secure the copies yourself.

◆ To provide to insurance companies. If a claim is disputed by your insurance company, a copy of your physician's records may help clarify the situation.

◆ To apply for disability or unemployment. Your attorney may need a copy of your medical records to better represent you during the review process.

◆ After you have been treated in a hospital or special clinic. Your primary treating physician will want to refer to the records kept by the hospital's health-care professionals.

Picture This/Lessons Learned

Picture This:

A person with fibromyalgia sees her physician each month for more than a year. After much deliberation, she decides that she can no longer continue to work and must file for disability. This individual discusses the situation with her physician, who agrees with the patient's decision and provides all the patient's records to the correct administrative office.

Neither the patient nor the health-care professional realized that there were multiple mistakes in the chart. A typist had misread the doctor's notes and the chart's cover letter noted that the patient only had 6 instead of 16 tender points. (Remember that 11 tender points are necessary for a diagnosis of fibromyalgia.) A letter from a previous physician was included in the chart that stated the patient seemed "stressed," and that all laboratory tests were negative. The physician had noted in the chart a comment that the patient made during her first appointment: "I just don't understand why I hurt all the time. Everyone says there is nothing wrong with me. Sometimes I don't think I can go on!" And then, finally, because the patient had so many symptoms to report to her doctor, there were times he got so involved in their conversation that he didn't note many of the important complaints.

The mistakes and misinterpretations contained in this chart will likely cause disability to be denied.

Lessons Learned:

It is important to review all aspects of your medical chart, especially if it is being shared with an individual or organization that is making a decision that will affect your treatment or future. Even if you have a supportive physician, it is important to review everything written in your chart yourself.

Although there are numerous situations in which it will be necessary or advantageous to request your medical records, there may be cases when you will not need to get personal copies.

Keeping Track of Medical Tests and Procedures

As with any chronic illness, it is important to keep track of the various tests and procedures that are performed by each health-care professional. Certain tests need to be repeated every few months, while others don't. By minimizing the number of tests that need to be repeated, you can reduce additional costs for you and your insurance company.

If you see multiple physicians, you may want to share test results instead of subjecting yourself to repetitive tests. If you accurately keep track of the tests and procedures you have already had, then you can easily provide a copy of the results to the specialist you are seeing, or ask the testing physician to forward the results to that other specialist.

For your convenience, a chart is provided in Appendix C to help you keep track of each test and procedure that you undergo. Make note of blood tests, trigger point injections, x-rays, MRIs, mammograms, colonoscopies, urine tests, bone density scans, and so on.

Tracking Health Insurance Claims

Ultimately, it is the responsibility of the patient to pay for any medical costs associated with medical services. If you have valid insurance (including Medicare or a state insurance program), you should present your card or information at the time that the medical services are rendered. Instead of being surprised when your insurance does not cover all the costs you incurred, make sure you are educated beforehand about your policy coverage. Do not be afraid to ask questions and speak to your insurance company prior to a doctor's appointment, hospitalization, procedure, or test.

Also, be sure that you completely understand the role your health-care professional will play in dealing with the insurance company. Some questions to ask the health-care professional (or the office staff) include ...

◆ Will your doctor's office get pre-authorization for certain tests, procedures, and surgeries, or are you responsible for that?

♦ Will your doctor accept the insurance company's payment as payment in full, or will you be responsible for the remaining amount?

♦ If you are having surgery, will there be other health-care professionals (for example, an anesthesiologist) involved in your care who will be billing you separately?

♦ Does your health-care provider submit your bills to the insurance company, or do you have to?

♦ Are you required to make a co-payment at the time of the appointment, or will your doctor bill you?

♦ If you go to the emergency room, will your insurance cover the cost of all the health-care professionals you see?

Obviously, there are many questions that you will need to address to be well informed about your particular situation and insurance coverage.

Pain Signal

Large medical bills will negatively impact the already difficult situation you are trying to deal with. If you do not feel up to getting the necessary pre-authorization form from your insurance company, or if you feel unable to negotiate your financial responsibilities with your treating physician, it is important to ask for help! A family member or friend may be better at acting as an advocate for you in these important matters. Just because you are sick when these administrative tasks must be taken care of, that doesn't mean you can put them off until you are feeling better. You must be sure that the financial matters related to your care are being dealt with in a timely, responsible manner.

If you are receiving medical care through a health maintenance organization (HMO) plan, there will be additional restrictions on which health-care professionals you can see, which treatments they will pre-authorize, and which they will disallow. You might even find that your HMO doctor has recommended treatments that were not approved by the HMO committee.

It is tempting to ignore the entire medical payment process and assume that the insurance company and doctors are handling everything satisfactorily. However, the reality is that you will receive a large bill from your medical provider for charges not covered under your insurance plan (including coverage that was reduced, denied, or disallowed).

The first step to understanding your insurance coverage is to get a written copy of the policy from your insurance company or your employer. Because most policy brochures are divided into separate sections, review the policy one subject at a time. This way you will not be overwhelmed when you first try to go through the policy. These sections might include ...

- **Eligibility.** This will tell you when your policy goes into effect.

- **Schedule of benefits.** This describes what the insurance company will pay and what you are responsible for.

- **Covered benefits.** This is a listing of what things are covered under the plan.

- **Claims procedures.** This tells you how to file a claim and how to appeal a denial.

- **Exclusions and limitations.** This lists the things that the plan does not cover. It also discusses which things are covered, but have special limits.

- **Definitions.** These define special terms and words used throughout the plan.

- **Termination of coverage.** This tells you when your coverage ends. It also includes a description of how you can get extended coverage under COBRA (Consolidated Omnibus Budget Reconciliation Act).

As you deal with making payments and filing insurance claims, be sure to document everything by taking detailed notes during the process. Make note of all telephone calls, in-person discussions with your physician's office staff, and so on. Keep copies of all correspondence, bills, receipts, and so on. Put all original letters and bills in a designated file folder or notebook. Make sure that you stay organized. If this task is too overwhelming for you, get help as soon as possible!

The following tips can help with filing insurance claims:

- Become educated about your condition.

- Know the terms of your insurance plan or your HMO policies.

- If you pay your own premiums, be sure you do it in a timely fashion. Some companies do offer a 30-day grace period, but if you are late with your payment, you may have your insurance discontinued.

- File your claims as soon as possible to avoid any mistakes, deadlines, or delays in payments. Check with your carrier to find out about pertinent deadlines.

- If your health-care professional is filing your claim, be sure that he or she has all your correct information. If you receive a bill from your physician telling you that he or she hasn't received payment from your insurance carrier, call your insurance company and follow up on the claim.

- Always verify that the medical procedures you are being charged for were actually performed. Check with your insurance company if you think you are being billed twice or overcharged.

Healthy Alternative
Make sure that you keep all notes and other information (letters, bills, receipts, and so on) in a file folder or notebook. Keep all documents for each claim together and well organized.

Finally, if you feel that you are being treated unfairly by your insurance carrier, seek professional legal help. Do not rush into a settlement if you feel that your expectations are not being met.

Changing Insurance Policies

There may be times in your life when you need to change your medical insurance. If you are not well informed before you make changes, you might end up without any medical insurance!

For example, if you change jobs, there are some important laws that will affect you. If you work for a company with 20 or more employees, you will be given an opportunity to continue your insurance through COBRA (Consolidated Omnibus Budget Reconciliation Act), which was passed by Congress in 1986 (www.cobrainsurance. com). COBRA contains provisions giving certain former employees and retirees (who were previously enrolled in their employer's health plan when they were working) the right to *temporarily* continue health coverage at group rates. COBRA coverage is usually more expensive than an employee's health coverage, because the former employee must pay the entire premium the employer used to pay. It is, however, usually less expensive than individual health coverage.

If you are eligible for COBRA benefits, you *must* notify your employer that you want to continue your benefits in writing *within 60 days* of the date you receive notice from your employer that you are eligible to continue your benefits. You have 45 days after electing coverage to pay the initial premium.

If you work for a company with fewer than 20 employees, you can continue your benefits for up to 12 months, but you must notify your employer in writing within 30 days of the date of your termination. This also applies if your work hours have been reduced to the point that you are no longer eligible for health insurance benefits. COBRA beneficiaries are usually eligible for group coverage for qualifying events for a maximum of 18 months due to termination or reduction in hours of work. Certain qualifying events may qualify a beneficiary to receive a maximum of 36 months of coverage.

The Least You Need to Know

- It is important to keep track of all medical records in your name and know how and when to get copies.

- The physician owns the medical chart, but the patient owns the information contained in the chart.

- Medical record policies are subject to a patchwork of state and federal laws and regulations. There is no continuity from state to state, but every health-care professional has a duty on the request of a patient (or the patient's representative) to release a copy of the record in a timely manner to the patient.

- Do not be afraid to ask questions and speak to your insurance company prior to a doctor's appointment, hospitalization, procedure, or test.

- File your claims as soon as possible to avoid any mistakes, deadlines, or delays in payments. Check with your carrier for the required deadlines.

- If you are not well informed about your medical insurance before you make changes, you may end up without any medical insurance!

Part 3

What Are the Treatment Options?

Although there isn't a cure for fibromyalgia or even a tried-and-true treatment protocol that works for everyone, there is a series of pharmacological and complementary alternatives that have been shown to help reduce many of the symptoms of fibromyalgia and its overlapping conditions. Just like many things in life, finding the answers to your questions may take time and patience, but the important thing is to recognize that you do have options. By evaluating them, deciding where your comfort level is, and then preceding with them in a step-by-step manner, you will achieve positive results.

To learn what options you have and how to make educated decisions, this part of the book gives you an extensive outline of the many treatment options that make up a multidisciplinary approach for treating fibromyalgia. From drugs that help alleviate symptoms, to lifestyle changes that can reduce stress and change the way you approach life, the options are many and the choices are yours.

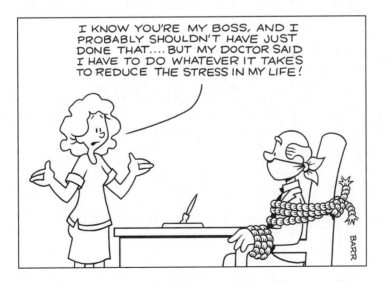

Chapter 9

Preparation for Treatment

In This Chapter

- ◆ Getting better one day at a time
- ◆ Finding the balance between patience and perseverance
- ◆ Discovering the multidisciplinary approach
- ◆ Discovering the interdisciplinary approach
- ◆ Finding the most successful treatments for you

Fibromyalgia is a complex illness. Just as you did research to learn more about fibromyalgia itself, you will need to do research about treatment options so you can select the treatments and approaches that will work best for you. Throughout the process of preparing for treatment—and even after you have started to be treated—you will want to stay up-to-date on new treatment options. Over the next few years, new pharmacological treatments specifically for fibromyalgia will be made available, new clinics that specialize in treating this illness will be established, and universities and hospitals will be creating facilities where multiple medical specialists will come together to ensure that patients receive coordinated care. In the meantime, you should become educated on your current options.

Getting Better Despite Chronic Illness

If you have never experienced a chronic illness before, you may think of a "treatment" as a process that has a beginning and an end. When I first became ill, my expectation was that I would go to a health-care professional, find out what was wrong, have a treatment prescribed (that had been proven to work and that would help me to get better), and then after the treatment I would be well once again. This had been my previous experience, whether I received antibiotics for an infection or had a broken arm put in a cast.

But fibromyalgia, like many other illnesses, is chronic. Treatments will ease and maybe even eliminate certain symptoms, but the illness itself has no end. These types of illnesses are treated with a combination of treatments individualized for each patient. And in the case of fibromyalgia, where there isn't any single, totally successful treatment (as of yet), it will be a process of trial and error.

With patience, you will get better—not all well—but much, much better. You can modify your lifestyle so that your symptoms very rarely get in the way of living your life fully. The focus of your life will be on something other than your fibromyalgia, and you will become a healthier and happier individual. It might take time, but just as I did, you can go from the depths of pain and misery to the realization of a new brighter, healthier, and happier life.

Picture This/Lessons Learned

Picture This:

In the mid-1990s my ability to participate in any physical activity was limited to walking to the mailbox each day and then falling back into bed exhausted and plagued with pain. After slowly reconditioning myself through yoga, water therapy, slow short walks, and then a routine on a treadmill, I can now ride a bike, hike in the mountains, and walk along the beach at sunset.

Lessons Learned:

When your health-care provider tells you to start exercising, don't panic! In the beginning, all you have to do is add some elements of activity to your day. If you slowly extend the amount of activity and eventually start stretching, then swimming, and then walking routinely, you will find yourself able to enjoy a much more active lifestyle.

Putting Together a Treatment Plan

When you are exploring the diverse number of treatment options that are presented for fibromyalgia on the Internet, in books, and even by various types of health-care providers, you may become overwhelmed by the huge number of options that are touted as beneficial. The sheer amount of information can make it difficult to determine which ones are *useful* and which ones will be helpful to *you*.

Although the self-management plan that you and your health-care team put together is individualized for you, today we know that some options have a higher success rate than others. We know that people with fibromyalgia are sensitive to medications, so the preferred treatment approach is one where both pharmacological and nonpharmacological interventions are used. Because the very nature of fibromyalgia involves multiple symptoms and overlapping conditions, a rehabilitation program that consists of biological, social, psychological, and spiritual approaches has proven to be the most effective.

We also know that, unfortunately, there are individuals and companies out there that claim to have a "cure." If there were a *cure*, there wouldn't be millions of people with fibromyalgia! Be aware of claims that seem too good to be true—because that's exactly what they are.

When it comes to treatment, you will try the things you feel most comfortable with and combine multiple treatments that will work together to improve not only your symptoms, but your overall functionality. It's a little bit like putting together a puzzle. There will be lots of individual pieces when you start, but as you put the pieces in place, the big picture will become recognizable and the pieces will come together with much less effort.

It is very important that you not become overwhelmed in the beginning. Just remember to take it a step at a time, a day at a time—and remember that there are options out there that will be helpful and will provide you with a better quality of life.

The Multidisciplinary Approach

In a multidisciplinary approach, the patient selects and utilizes the expertise of different specialists who practice both traditional and nontraditional medical approaches. Unlike a common illness such as a bacterial infection (where we know that the root cause of the illness is a harmful type of bacteria), fibromyalgia involves multiple neuroendocrine abnormalities, but the exact root cause is not yet fully understood. Therefore, the multidisciplinary approach tries multiple ways to help decrease or eliminate the many symptoms and overlapping conditions that make up fibromyalgia syndrome. Even more importantly, the treatments are designed to increase your functionality and quality of life. In other words, you may still have to deal with some of the symptoms of fibromyalgia, but you can find ways to reduce their overall impact on your life and their severity should decrease over time.

It may sound trite, but fibromyalgia can help you learn things that will enable you to become a more balanced individual. Living a balanced life can be viewed as a *treatment*. Some of the key lessons that you can learn from having fibromyalgia—including patience and perseverance, maintaining a positive attitude while being willing to accept reality, and living life practically and purposefully—can actually help reduce your symptoms. As your priorities change, you will become a more balanced individual and find you can develop and accept new ways to approach life that will help you improve both physically and emotionally.

def•i•ni•tion

A **treatment** for fibromyalgia is an approach (or an intervention) that is likely to improve a patient's symptoms. The goal of treatment is to help people with fibromyalgia better manage their symptoms.

It is up to you. You can find strength from this illness or you can let it get the best of you. Until better treatments are developed (which we all hope will be in the near future), you have to find the patience and perseverance to discern which treatments are of help to you.

Currently, most individuals receive treatment from a variety of health specialists who have expertise in a range of health disciplines. A self-management approach involves a partnership between you and a team of health-care providers. Your personal self-management plan will include a multidisciplinary approach to treatment. In other words, you will evaluate which treatment options are most suited to your needs and then implement them in combination with one another. You should maintain control of your overall treatment, while basing your decisions on the advice of your health-care team. Today, we know that an effective self-management program for fibromyalgia should include the following:

- Physical fitness
- Sleep retraining
- Medication management
- *Psychosocial support*

- Fatigue management
- Flare management
- Pain management

def•i•ni•tion

Psychosocial support refers to the avenues that are available to a person with fibromyalgia as well as family and caregivers who help them with emotional issues and provide supportive services. These resources should be an integral part of their care and support and can include counseling, support groups, and community services.

From Multidisciplinary to the Interdisciplinary Approach

In a multidisciplinary approach, patients decide which specialists are going to become a part of their health-care team. The patient evaluates (along with the advice of the health-care professionals) which medical treatment options are desired and affordable. This places much of the responsibility on the person with fibromyalgia, and can result in fragmented care that is expensive. If you are seeing multiple doctors, the lack of coordination might impede the amount of benefit you receive. However, if you can arrange for cooperation and teamwork between the health-care professionals you are seeing, you should be able to minimize fragmented care.

To respond to this problem of fragmented care, doctors, clinics, and universities have tried to incorporate a variety of specialties into *interdisciplinary programs* that can provide coordinated and concurrent care for the patient. The interdisciplinary health-care team sees the patient in a setting where multiple health-care professionals have come together at one facility to help in a collaborative manner.

def•i•ni•tion

In an **interdisciplinary program** or approach, the patient's health needs are addressed by a group of collaborating health-care professionals who specialize in a variety of health-care disciplines. Because researchers are still looking for effective treatment modalities for fibromyalgia, the goal of the interdisciplinary approach is to help the patient focus on managing the illness by establishing realistic expectations and learning management techniques.

In the case of fibromyalgia, the emphasis in this type of setting is on education. Treatment must involve not only the relief of symptoms (because some symptoms cannot be completely relieved), but must also focus on changing patients' perceptions of their illness and helping them develop behaviors to better cope. Because one of the best ways to improve the chances of symptom reduction is through the development of coping skills, interdisciplinary programs help teach participants ways to change negative health behaviors. They also teach how to develop positive outcomes through personal attitude changes. Another aspect of this type of program is the reliance on the group dynamic. Studies have shown that people who have an active social network live longer. This type of program allows the individual to take part in group interactions, which provide support and help to eliminate isolationism.

Because of the cost involved in creating interdisciplinary centers, only a limited number of such programs have been developed. The need is great, however, and new clinics are being established to meet it.

The majority of fibromyalgia treatment centers that exist today, however, implement their own specific treatment philosophy. Although multiple health-care professionals come together to offer their expertise, the centers usually only implement treatments that fall into one category of treatment.

Healthy Alternative

Many of the fibromyalgia treatment centers that exist today focus on alternative treatment approaches. Participation in these types of programs might include the use of treatments such as acupuncture, massage, exercise in the form of yoga or Tai Chi, meditation, and the use of supplements. Other types of treatment options are not part of the program.

If there isn't an interdisciplinary clinic near you, talk to your doctor and ask for health-care professional referrals. Often a rheumatologist will be familiar with other specialists who could become a part of your health-care team. You can also get referrals from your local fibromyalgia support group or national organizations such as the National Headache Foundation, the American Sleep Apnea Association, the American Pain Association, the American Academy of Pain Management, and the National Fibromyalgia Association. An extensive list of these organizations is included in Appendix B.

Deciding Which Treatments Are Right for You

An illness that has multiple symptoms, such as fibromyalgia, requires multiple treatments. These treatments may be provided by several different health-care providers. The most common specialists who can improve the symptoms and functionality in a person with fibromyalgia include (but the list is not limited to) the following:

- Internists
- Rheumatologists
- Neurologists
- Pain-management specialists
- Acupuncturists
- Massage therapists
- Water therapists
- Physical therapists

- Occupational therapists
- Psychologists
- Psychiatrists
- Nutritional specialists
- Sleep therapists
- Physiatrists
- Physical medicine and rehabilitation specialists

While several different providers may provide you with treatment, all treatments need to be reviewed by your primary health-care provider, because everything you take or do can interact with other treatments and can impact the decisions of your doctor. Just because you have been taking a certain medication for sleep does not mean that it will always be appropriate or necessary. Likewise, you might need new treatments or can reduce or stop treatments as your symptoms wax and wane.

Always be sure that your primary health-care professional is apprised of every treatment you try. If you are open about the treatment decisions you have made outside of your doctor's care, you will be better informed about what effects these practices will have on your overall health—and your health-care professional will be able to make better decisions on how to treat you, because he or she will have all the facts.

Fast Fact

According to the *American Family Physician,* "Physicians should spend some time eliciting and hearing the ongoing narrative of the struggle of living with a chronic disease and attempt to ameliorate the effects of the symptoms on the patient's quality of life. Ideally, the practitioner will collaborate with the patient to construct a unique treatment plan consonant with the patient's circumstances. That plan will necessarily evolve within the context of the physician-patient relationship."

Starting Treatment

As mentioned, research continues to provide information to help us better understand which treatment options appear to be the most beneficial to people with fibromyalgia.

It makes sense to start your treatment program with those interventions that have the highest percentage of success. Several of the most well-known fibromyalgia specialists have provided their thoughts on the subject:

Don L. Goldenberg, M.D., professor of medicine at Tufts University School of Medicine, and chief of rheumatology, Newton-Wellesley Hospital, Massachusetts, treats the pain and fatigue that his patients experience in a multidisciplinary fashion. He feels education is the key to empower his patients. Initially he likes to focus on diagnosing and treating primary sleep disturbances, reducing stress through cognitive behavioral techniques, and utilizing a physical therapist and a doctor of physical medicine and rehabilitation. Medications that he finds helpful to people with fibromyalgia are analgesics, low doses of sleep medications, and low doses of antidepressants that have an effect on multiple fibromyalgia symptoms. Dr. Goldenberg looks forward to new medications being developed that will help eliminate the sluggish response in the hypothalamic-pituitary-adrenal systems of the fibromyalgia patient.

Robert Bennett, M.D., F.R.C.P., professor of medicine, Oregon Health Sciences University (OHSU) and retired chairman of the Arthritis and Rheumatic Disease Program, Portland, Oregon, notes that the main complaint of people with fibromyalgia is pain. His research has shown that Ultram (tramadol) and Ultracet (tramadol plus Tylenol) are the most useful pain medications for patients with widespread body pain, because they work on the central nervous system. For local pain that involves multiple areas of tenderness in muscles—which are called myofascial trigger points—he suggests the use of myofascial trigger-point injections and spray and stretch.

Mark J. Pellegrino, M.D., is board certified in physical medicine and rehabilitation and electrodiagnostic medicine, and has authored numerous books on fibromyalgia. Dr. Pellegrino, himself diagnosed with fibromyalgia, is aware that many people with fibromyalgia are sensitive to medications and can experience side effects. Nevertheless, he feels that medications can provide great benefits to relieve pain, improve sleep, and improve mood. He suggests that the patient and doctor experiment to determine which medications help best control symptoms.

Muhammad B. Yunus, M.D., is a board-certified rheumatologist, a fibromyalgia researcher, and a professor of medicine at the University of Illinois, Peoria. Dr. Yunus states that the treatment of a fibromyalgia patient should begin with a physician who possesses empathy and a willingness to listen and help. He believes that education, assurance, and an understanding attitude of the treating physician are important aspects of treatment. He emphasizes nondrug treatments first, such as sleep hygiene, patient self-responsibility, and gradually increasing physical exercise. He finds periodic injections of tender or trigger points with a local anesthetic very useful. He uses a multidisciplinary approach, referring patients to an appropriate specialist as needed.

Stuart L. Silverman, M.D., clinical professor of medicine at UCLA, has been the medical director of the Fibromyalgia Rehab Program at Cedars-Sinai Medical Center for the past 10 years. The Fibromyalgia Rehab Program is an interdisciplinary group rehabilitation program in Los Angeles, California. Dr. Silverman points out that self-management empowers people with fibromyalgia to make changes in their health behaviors (such as learning to exercise regularly, to eat well, and to manage pain and flares), reduces symptoms of fibromyalgia, and improves function. People with fibromyalgia need a slow, gradual program that will not result in painful flares. The Cedars-Sinai program emphasizes self-efficacy that develops confidence that patients can change their health behaviors, manage pain, and get better. He stresses the importance of helping people with fibromyalgia to hope and believe that they can get well.

Most doctors encourage you to become educated about your treatment options so you can better understand what your health-care professionals are recommending. This will ensure that you are better informed to make decisions and, if necessary, to search out the specialists you want to consult with.

Remember that your ultimate goal is hardiness—in other words, working toward your own personal best—and ensuring a healthier lifestyle, which can also reduce your body's overall hypersensitivity to pain and fatigue. Whatever treatment you and your doctor decide to pursue, it is important that you move away from *thinking about* doing something that will improve your health—and start *doing it*.

The Least You Need to Know

- The preferred treatment approach for fibromyalgia is one in which both pharmacological and nonpharmacological interventions are used.

- Because the very nature of fibromyalgia involves multiple symptoms and overlapping conditions, a rehabilitation program made up of biological, social, psychological, and spiritual approaches has proven to be the most effective.

◆ In a multidisciplinary approach, the patient selects and utilizes the expertise of different specialists who practice both traditional and nontraditional medical approaches.

◆ It makes sense to start your treatment program with those interventions that have the highest success rate.

◆ In an interdisciplinary approach, the patient works with a group of health-care professionals who represent a variety of specialties. They focus on a collaborative approach to help patients learn how to better cope with their illness.

Pharmacological Medications

In This Chapter

- ◆ Understanding off-label medications
- ◆ Using medications for pain
- ◆ Using medications for anxiety and muscle relaxation
- ◆ Using medications for sleeplessness
- ◆ Helping reduce pain through trigger-point injections

Only a few years ago the idea of a medication specifically approved for fibromyalgia seemed impossible, something that might only be a dream for the distant future. However, on June 21, 2007, the Food and Drug Administration (FDA) approved Lyrica as the first medication for the treatment of fibromyalgia. Several comprehensive research studies were done to look at the drug's safety, how it was tolerated, and how well it worked on reducing fibromyalgia symptoms. Laboratory tests showed that about 30 percent of fibromyalgia patients on Lyrica compared to those on placebo experienced relief of their symptoms, including pain. Lyrica is the first of several medications that the FDA is checking for approval in fibromyalgia. Many pharmaceutical companies are in the process of researching other compounds with the specific purpose of alleviating fibromyalgia symptoms.

There is great optimism held by fibromyalgia researchers that treating doctors finally have scientifically proven medications to help relieve fibromyalgia symptoms. The dream has become a reality, and while we wait for more FDA authorizations, there are many medications that can be prescribed off-label to treat the symptoms of this illness. It is important to understand that even Lyrica, which received specific approval as a medication for fibromyalgia, does not cure the problem but rather helps relieve symptoms. Because a person with fibromyalgia may suffer from numerous symptoms, it is important for you and your health-care professional to discuss which symptoms are the most severe and need to be treated with a prescribed medication. Together you will want to evaluate their safety and how effective you find them in helping to alleviate your specific problems.

This chapter discusses various drug treatment options that have been found to benefit people with fibromyalgia. With the exception of Lyrica, they all come under the heading of off-label prescriptions. Doctors have successfully determined the efficacy of drugs on their own and built up a community of knowledge concerning the use of existing medications to treat fibromyalgia. Although not everyone finds these medications to be helpful, through a process of trial and error, you and your health-care professional should be able to find ways to treat your symptoms with existing pharmacological agents.

Off-Label Treatments

As fibromyalgia research expands, it will eventually provide us with a better understanding of the cause(s) of this illness. Armed with this knowledge, pharmaceutical companies will be able to develop and gain approval for more medications that will be designed specifically to treat those causes. As new prescriptions become available, health-care professionals can try them for symptom relief, but a combination of new drugs and off-label medications will probably still be necessary to improve a person's quality of life and to relieve chronic pain.

Patients must rely on their health-care professional's knowledge about existing medications that have the ability to relieve symptoms similar to those that exist in other conditions. For example, pain, fatigue, muscle spasms, sleep disturbances, and so on are some of these symptoms. Even though the medications that are prescribed to fibromyalgia patients aren't approved for treating fibromyalgia, your health-care professional has the legal right to prescribe any medication for any reason he or she sees fit. For example, selective serotonin reuptake inhibitors (SSRIs), which were initially developed to relieve depression, are now commonly prescribed for patients with fibromyalgia because they help reduce pain, improve sleep, and improve mood. Without the ability to prescribe *off-label* medications, patients with illnesses for which there are no standard treatments would have no pharmacological help.

def•i•ni•tion

The term **off-label** refers to a legal practice in which physicians prescribe a drug approved by the Food and Drug Administration (FDA) for a use that is not approved. That could mean prescribing a dosage higher or lower than the FDA-approved dosage; at a different interval than the FDA-approved interval; or for a condition for which the FDA has not approved the drug. Virtually every person with this illness that has taken medication has been treated with an off-label prescription.

Although off-label treatments may sound dangerous, the American Medical Association strongly supports doctors' rights to prescribe FDA-approved drugs for any reasons that they believe are helpful. The system works because health-care professionals are making decisions based on their extensive knowledge of science and what's in the patient's best interest. The system would work even better if the patients were also aware of ways to help protect themselves.

Healthy Alternative

To better protect yourself when taking off-label medications, be sure to do the following:

Discuss in detail with your health-care professional the risks associated with taking the medication.

Don't take something that is so new that the use is still very controversial.

Be an informed consumer. Take the time to research what is being said about the medication in books, magazines, and on the Internet.

Consulting with Your Physician

When you consult with your physician about possible pharmacological treatments, it is important that you understand what he or she is prescribing and why. I have spoken to many people with fibromyalgia who are taking medications that they are unfamiliar with and aren't even sure why they are taking the medications! Never take a medication that you have not discussed at length with your health-care professional. Remember that people with fibromyalgia can be sensitive to medications, so whenever you try a new medication, take the time to discuss the dosage level with your health-care professional. Let your physician know immediately if you are experiencing any side effects or unusual new symptoms. Even if you aren't sure if what you are experiencing is a side effect, it is better to alert your physician and be safe rather than sorry. Never feel intimidated by your physician. If you are uncomfortable taking a specific medication, let your health-care professional know about your concerns. If you have additional questions about a certain medication that has been prescribed for you, talk to your pharmacist. They are extremely knowledgeable about the uses of certain medications and their side effects.

Treating the Pain

The following sections discuss how you can treat the pain.

Antidepressants

Often when a health-care professional suggests an antidepressant to treat the symptoms of fibromyalgia, the patient gets concerned that the physician thinks that they are just depressed. In reality, antidepressants are often prescribed to treat multiple symptoms, including pain and sleep disturbances. If an antidepressant is prescribed for you, don't take offense; instead talk to your health-care professional and find out why he or she is suggesting that you take an antidepressant. One fibromyalgia researcher explained to me that if the medical field had known all of the things that antidepressants are capable of treating, they would have never been called antidepressants in the first place!

In the 1980s, the initial research on fibromyalgia reported low *serotonin* levels in people with this disorder. Therefore, the original pharmacological approaches (that are still being used today) for treating fibromyalgia include amitriptyline, cyclobenzaprine, and other tricyclic antidepressants. These drugs tend to increase serotonin throughout the central nervous system. Studies have found that amitriptyline is effective in decreasing pain intensity, improving sleep quality, and reducing general fibromyalgia symptom severity. Cyclobenzaprine seems to have more consistent improvement in ratings of sleep than in pain intensity. The tricyclic medicines are effective, but frequent side effects include dry mouth, weight gain, and drowsiness.

def•i•ni•tion

Serotonin is a neurotransmitter (a chemical messenger) that is produced in the brain and facilitates the passage of impulses from one neuron (nerve cell) to the next across the small gaps between neurons, called synapses. Serotonin, which is found in the intestinal wall, blood vessels, and central nervous system, is known to influence the functioning of the cardiovascular, renal, immune, and gastrointestinal systems. It is known to modulate mood, emotions, sleep, and appetite.

Selective serotonin reuptake inhibitors such as Prozac, Zoloft, Paxil, Effexor, Serzone, and Celexa are effective in improving mood and decreasing pain. Studies have shown that both medications have helped patients with sleep, mood, and even fatigue complaints.

Recent studies have indicated that patients with fibromyalgia may have *norepinephrine-evoked* pain. This finding supports the hypothesis that fibromyalgia may be a sympathetically maintained pain syndrome. Scientists have recently initiated studies on medications that work on both serotonin and norepinephrine with good results, including the development of Cymbalta and Milnacipran for the treatment of fibromyalgia.

def•i•ni•tion _____

> **Norepinephrine** is a neurotransmitter (a chemical messenger) that mediates chemical communication in the sympathetic nervous system, a branch of the autonomic nervous system. Like other neurotransmitters, it is released at synaptic nerve endings to transmit the signal from a nerve cell to other cells. It increases heart rate as well as blood pressure and helps mobilize the body's resources to meet stressful situations.

Cymbalta (duloxetine), another medication that recently received approval for the treatment of fibromyalgia by the FDA, inhibits the reuptake of both serotonin and norepinephrine. It is part of a new class of drugs known as Norepinephrine Serotonin Reuptake Inhibitors or NSRIs. Cymbalta was developed as an antidepressant but it is also used as a medication to relieve painful diabetic neuropathy. Research on fibromyalgia symptoms have yielded results that demonstrate measurable improvement in approximately 30 percent of study participants compared to a placebo. Research has shown that Cymbalta administered at 60 mg twice a day was found to be effective on most outcome measures, including pain, particularly in women, and was safe and well tolerated. Side effects include insomnia, dry mouth, and constipation, but were not common in all participants of the studies.

Milnacipran is another NSRI medication currently under FDA scrutiny for approval in the treatment of fibromyalgia symptoms. In scientific studies, Milnacipran-treated patients showed significant improvements in pain, fatigue, and mood compared to those who received a placebo. It was found efficacious in approximately 30 percent of study participants in treating pain and other fibromyalgia symptoms at both 100 mg and 200 mg daily doses. Nausea was the most common side effect.

Antidepressants venlafaxine and nefazodone are medications that also inhibit the reuptake of both serotonin and norepinephrine.

It is not surprising that a person challenged with chronic pain might become unhappy or even develop depression. However, both the disease itself and depression are based on neurochemistry, such as low serotonin. By using antidepressants, the individual benefits not only because antidepressants are useful in treating pain and sleep problems, but also because they are effective in treating depression and anxiety. Note, however, that the dose for treating depression is greater than the dose for treating pain or improving sleep.

Anticonvulsants

Lyrica, approved by the FDA for the treatment of fibromyalgia, is considered to be an anticonvulsant-type medication that can be used to treat neuropathic pain or pain that is generated by the nerves themselves. Individuals with fibromyalgia have been shown to experience pain differently from other people. Studies have shown that such patients have decreased pain after taking Lyrica, but the mechanism by which Lyrica produces such an effect is unknown. Two double-blind, controlled clinical trials, involving about 1,800 patients, support approval for use in treating fibromyalgia with doses of 450 milligrams per day. Lyrica already was approved for treating partial seizures, pain following the rash of shingles, and pain associated with diabetes nerve damage (diabetic neuropathy). Some of Lyrica's side effects include weight gain, mild-to-moderate dizziness, and sleepiness. Studies indicated that the side effects seem to be related to the amount of medication taken. It can also impair motor function and cause problems with concentration and attention. You should only use this medication if it is prescribed for you by your health-care professional, and any adverse effects should be reported immediately.

The scientific studies conducted on Lyrica demonstrated that doses of 450 mg per day seem to work as well as 600 mg. This medication was titrated a little at a time, which seemed to help people tolerate its side effects. Research investigations have shown that it is efficacious in about 30 percent of fibromyalgia patients.

Anticonvulsant-type medications often work best on patients who have symptoms of burning or hot electric shock feelings, especially in their hands and feet. They may find relief with antiseizure medicines that help treat neuropathic pain. Besides Lyrica, these medicines include Neurontin, Dilantin, Depakote, and Tegretol. Studies on Neurontin in the treatment of fibromyalgia are underway and preliminary results look promising. The outcome data from these studies will help determine the correct dosages of Neurontin for people with fibromyalgia, which are currently administered at between 100 and 3,000 milligrams per day. This medication has a sedating effect, so if your health-care professional suggests Neurontin, you will want to discuss what dosage is appropriate for you.

Dopamine Agonists

A study published by Andrew Holman, M.D., demonstrated that Mirapex (pramipexole), a dopamine agonist commonly used for Parkinson's disease, works well for some people with fibromyalgia. Dopamine agonists directly stimulate the receptors in nerves in the brain that normally would be stimulated by dopamine. Often people with fibromyalgia suffer from restless legs syndrome, which is commonly experienced at night during sleep. In the study, the dose was slowly titrated to 4.5 mg taken at bedtime. It was generally well tolerated by the patients in the study, but nausea was a major side effect. To counteract this problem, antinausea medication was used during the titrating period with good effect.

Another common side effect is the sudden onset of sleepiness. Again, it is imperative that you work closely with your health-care professional when you begin a medication protocol and be sure to report any adverse side effects you might experience. Decreased pain was the most pronounced benefit of Mirapex in this study. Further research is now being done to see if the results can be duplicated. Mirapex and Requip (ropinirole) are the newest dopamine agonists and may cause fewer side effects than the older dopamine agonists (such as bromocriptine).

Not only is pain the main symptom of fibromyalgia, but it is a symptom that can be treated in a variety of different ways and with a variety of different types of medications. Because people with fibromyalgia have different types of pain, your health-care professional might prescribe different kinds of medications. All of your pain may seem similar but your physician will determine what type you are experiencing and what treatment will be best suited to help alleviate it.

Pain has different causes, such as inflammation, tissue or bone injury, neurological abnormalities, and so on; therefore, the treatment will be different depending on its cause. Fibromyalgia pain is neurological in nature, but people with fibromyalgia can suffer with other types of pain, too.

Not only are there different medications for different kinds of pain, but there are also different dosages that can be helpful when pain varies. At times you may have to adjust your medications depending on the level of pain you are experiencing at that particular time. For example, the dosage of Ultram (tramadol) can vary greatly. Your health-care professional might suggest that you take 50 mg twice a day, but when your pain is more severe he or she could increase the dosage up to 50 mg four or six times a day. Pain can also affect other symptoms. If you are experiencing high levels of pain, you might also begin to suffer from anxiety or sleeplessness. Many of the medications that you take will have an effect on more than one symptom.

Nonsteroidal Anti-Inflammatory Drugs

Anti-inflammatory medicines include aspirin; nonsteroidal anti-inflammatories (NSAIDs) such as ibuprofen, Naprosyn, Lodine, and Daypro; the newer group of medications referred to as Cox-II inhibitors, such as Celebrex; and corticosteroids such as prednisone and dexamethasone. These medications provide two benefits: they act as anti-inflammatory agents and pain relievers. Some of these medicines, such as ibuprofen, are available both over the counter and by prescription. Because fibromyalgia does not involve *inflammation*, these drugs may be less effective. If the NSAIDs are helpful for overall fibromyalgia pain, they can be continued on a regular basis as long as there are no major side effects, such as stomach irritation. Unless the person with fibromyalgia also has an inflammatory illness (such as lupus, rheumatoid arthritis, osteoarthritis, and so on), corticosteroids, which treat inflammation, usually prove to be counterproductive.

def•i•ni•tion

Inflammation occurs in autoimmune illnesses such as rheumatoid arthritis, inflammatory bowel diseases, lupus, and scleroderma. It is the first response of the immune system to infection or irritation and is characterized by redness, heat, swelling, pain, and dysfunction of the organs involved. Although at one time fibromyalgia was thought to be inflammatory, we now know that it is not.

So why does an anti-inflammatory such as ibuprofen help fibromyalgia, if fibromyalgia is not an inflammatory illness? Pain relievers such as ibuprofen work with your cells, your body's nerve endings, and your brain to keep you from feeling the pain. When you take a pain reliever such as ibuprofen, it keeps the cells from making and releasing a chemical called prostaglandin. When the cells don't release this substance, it means the brain won't receive the pain message as quickly or clearly.

Analgesics

Analgesics are medications that treat pain. They can be over-the-counter medicines such as aspirin and acetaminophen, or prescription-strength pain pills such as narcotics (opiates), codeine, Vicodin, Darvocet, OxyContin, and Percocet. Ultram (tramadol) and Ultracet (tramadol and acetaminophen) are non-narcotic pain-relieving medications. These medications do not alter fibromyalgia, but they can help take the edge off pain.

A study conducted in 2003 by Robert M. Bennett, M.D., a pain specialist at the Oregon Health and Science University, and published in the *American Journal of Medicine* compared Ultracet (37.5 mg tramadol hydrochloride/325 mg acetaminophen tablets) to a placebo in 315 fibromyalgia patients. Patients who used Ultracet experienced significantly better pain relief than those who received the placebo.

Narcotics

Narcotic analgesics act on the central nervous system to relieve pain. The use of these medications, especially for fibromyalgia, continues to be debated throughout the medical and patient communities.

Dr. Robert Bennett believes that narcotics should not be the first line of defense against pain and that "opioids should be used sparingly"; however, he feels that they should not be withheld if other analgesics have failed. His experience has been that his fibromyalgia patients want to try opiates but then give them up because of their side effects (nausea, dizziness, constipation, and tiredness). He also points out that addiction to opioids is not typical among persons with fibromyalgia.

Fast Fact

Kim Jones, Ph.D., Oregon Health and Science University (OHSU), who has hosted web-based chats on Web MD, recommends that if other pain medications have not been successful, you might consider taking short-acting narcotics such as Lortab or Vicodin.

Some health-care professionals recommend using opiates on a very limited basis to help relieve more intense pain that occurs during a flare-up of symptoms; yet others believe that the use of narcotics in the treatment of fibromyalgia is dangerous and never warranted. In the medical literature on the subject, the consensus seems to be that only about 5 to 10 percent of people with fibromyalgia are taking narcotics to treat their pain.

OxyContin, MS Contin, and methadone are longer-acting narcotics. Anne Winkler, M.D., medical director of the Fibromyalgia Program at the Smith-Glynn-Callaway Medical facility in Springfield, Missouri, believes that if a long-acting narcotic is used, it should be OxyContin, because she feels there is less chance for patient addiction. However, she points out that the use of opioids for people with fibromyalgia should be a last resort.

Treating the Pain and More!

There are times when pain can be decreased in a person with fibromyalgia by treating the secondary symptoms of anxiety, muscle spasms, and sleep disturbances. We know that pain can be aggravated when you are dealing with multiple symptoms or when overlapping conditions are also causing you distress. For example, if your sleep is disturbed and you are lying in bed tossing and turning, it is not surprising that your body might experience more pain. Or if you are anxious and experiencing tightness and spasms in your muscles, a common experience can be more pain in these affected areas of your body. It can be helpful to treat these additional symptoms with symptom-specific medications, which will also help provide relief from your bodywide fibromyalgia pain.

Antianxiety Medications

Even though a medication is referred to in a particular category such as antianxiety medications, you must realize that these medications can be prescribed for more than one reason. Various medicines, including antidepressants and muscle relaxants, are used to treat anxiety and pain. Benzodiazepines, such as Klonopin, Ativan, and Xanax are effective in reducing anxiety, which can be a problem for people with fibromyalgia because it contributes to pain, muscle tension, sleeplessness, and irritability. Because these medicines do cause sedation, they can also be used to improve sleep, especially when the individual is experiencing leg symptoms (such as pain, restless legs syndrome, and jerking of the legs called myoclonus) that interfere with sleep.

Low-dose Klonopin therapy is one way to enhance the inhibitory function of GABA and the excitatory receptors (MMDA) in the central nervous system.

Muscle Relaxants

Muscle relaxants can be prescribed to help decrease pain in people with fibromyalgia. Medications in this classification include Flexeril, Soma, Skelaxin, and Robaxin. Dr. Mark Pellegrino says that these medications do not seem to actually decrease muscle spasms or truly relax muscles, because the painful area still has detectable spasms. Instead, the medicine appears to help by a central neurologic mechanism that reduces muscle pain.

Drowsiness can be a side effect, so these medicines should only be taken at a time when they won't interfere with driving or concentration. Flexeril is a popular medicine for people with fibromyalgia to take at night to help with pain and sleep.

The antispasticity category of medicines can be used to treat muscle spasms. Two of these medications, Zanaflex and baclofen, have been shown to help reduce back muscle spasms and pain. Antispasticity medicines are primarily intended for people who have neurological conditions causing involuntary muscle spasms (such as spinal cord injuries, multiple sclerosis, or strokes). However, these medicines might be able to help fibromyalgia patients who experience numerous muscle spasms.

Sleep Medications

Medications that treat sleep disturbances and have already been discussed include analgesics, antidepressants, and muscle relaxants. True sleep modifiers, however, include benzodiazepines such as Restoril and hypnotic nonbenzodiazepines such as Ambien. The most commonly reported concern about using sleep modifiers, especially benzodiazepams, is that they have a potential habit-forming effect. Ambien is reported by physicians to be less habit-forming than other sleep modifiers, but it can cause rebound insomnia when it's stopped. Sonata is a newer sleep modifier that is not habit-forming.

Xyrem (sodium oxybate), approved by the FDA as a medication for narcolepsy, is another type of sleep compound that is currently being studied for the treatment of fibromyalgia. It assists people in reaching REM or stage 3 and 4 sleep, which helps with the production of growth hormone, known to be low in many fibromyalgia patients. Preliminary study results are promising, so watch for news about this remarkable medication. People in the studies reported no "hangover" effect with Xyrem, and their pain improved as did many of their other symptoms.

Sleep modifiers are short-acting so they work to improve deep sleep during the night, while allowing you to feel more rested and alert by morning. Although these medications are often prescribed for a short period of time, people with fibromyalgia, under the strict care of a health-care professional, may continue to take these medications for extended time periods.

Pain Signal

Sleep disturbances can be specific and nonspecific. If the problem is nonspecific, sleep-modifying medications may improve your quality of sleep. However, if the problem is specific, such as sleep apnea, restless legs syndrome, or nocturnal bruxism (nighttime teeth grinding), the treatments vary and sleep modifiers may not be enough to improve sleep. To know what is affecting your sleep, it is helpful to be evaluated at a sleep clinic or sleep laboratory.

Trigger-Point Injections

For treating localized *myofascial pain*, such as the muscles in the neck or shoulders, a series of trigger-point injections might bring temporary pain relief. Although there are a variety of medications that can be used in this treatment, 1 to 2 percent procaine or lidocaine (local anesthetics) is usually preferred. Injections using Botox (a botulinum toxin) have recently been found to help temporarily reduce localized pain and migraine headaches.

def•i•ni•tion

Myofascial pain is caused by "trigger points," sensitive and painful areas between the muscle and fascia. Symptoms can range from referred pain through myofascial trigger points to specific pains in other areas of the body. The precise cause of myofascial pain is not fully understood and is undergoing research in several medical fields.

If you are to receive a trigger-point injection treatment, make sure your health-care professional can accurately identify the trigger-point location and is well experienced in performing these injections. This will help ensure that the injections will not create adverse side effects. Dr. Robert Bennett suggests that by performing "myofascial spray and stretch" techniques, your physician can often enhance the benefit of the trigger-point injections. Spray and stretch consists of applying a vapo-coolant spray, such as ethyl chloride, on the skin over the trigger point while performing a passive stretch of the muscle.

Your Notes and Questions on Pharmacological Treatments

Now that you have read an overview of some of the pharmacological treatment options for people with fibromyalgia, take some time to make notes and to develop questions for your health-care professional. Remember that none of these medications have been specifically approved for the treatment of fibromyalgia. They are used because research points to certain physiological abnormalities, such as low levels of serotonin, or through trial and error the medical community has found certain medications to be useful in reducing symptoms. It is important that you understand the reasons why your health-care professional has prescribed certain medications and what the risks are associated with taking that particular medication.

The Least You Need to Know

◆ Today, Lyrica has been approved by the FDA as a treatment for fibromyalgia. Several other medications are being scrutinized by the FDA as potential drugs for fibromyalgia and should be approved shortly.

◆ Analgesics are medications that treat pain. They can be over-the-counter medicines such as aspirin and acetaminophen, or prescription-strength pain pills such as narcotics (opiates), codeine, Vicodin, Darvocet, OxyContin, and Percocet.

◆ Norepinephrine Serotonin Reuptake Inhibitors or NSRIs, a new class of medications, are showing promise in the treatment of fibromyalgia. Cymbalta and Milnacipran are two of these medications waiting for FDA approval.

◆ Fibromyalgia patients who have symptoms of burning or hot electric shock feelings, especially in their hands and feet, may find relief with antiseizure medicines that help treat neuropathic pain.

◆ Sleep modifiers are short-acting so they work to improve deep sleep during the night, while allowing you to feel more rested and alert by morning.

◆ For treating localized myofascial pain, such as the muscles in the neck or shoulders, a series of trigger-point injections may bring temporary pain relief.

Chapter 11

Complementary, Alternative, and Integrative Therapies

In This Chapter

- Defining complementary, alternative, and integrative therapies

- Explaining acupuncture, massage, chiropractic manipulation, physical therapy (PT), aquatic therapy, and occupational therapy (OT)

- Discussing yoga, Tai Chi, Pilates, supplements, herbs, and electro-magnetic therapy

- Understanding medical alternatives

It wasn't too long ago that we went to our family doctor whenever we were sick and whatever he recommended was a "prescription for wellness." Today we have many more choices. Not only can we see a so-called Western medical doctor specializing in a specific medicine (family practice, rheumatology, osteopathy, neurology), but alternative or complementary practices are now also available and accepted as legitimate options. As the use of complementary therapies becomes more popular, and Western health-care professionals begin to recommend massage, acupuncture, supplements, and so on to their patients, each of us will need a better understanding of these options to decide what is most beneficial for our overall health.

In this chapter, you learn more about the alternative and complementary treatments that are used to help people with fibromyalgia. You will also come to understand that our health-care system is changing because of the needs of people with illnesses, such as fibromyalgia, that do not respond well to a pharmacological approach alone. As health-care professionals begin to recognize the benefits of these types of treatment options, our medical community will have to find ways to help patients coordinate these options into their pursuit of better health. Today the patient must take responsibility in coordinating both Western and Eastern medicine practices. However, it won't be long before the concept of intertwining the two becomes more accepted and the number of clinics that provide an integrated approach will increase.

Integrative Medicine

To understand which treatments are best to reduce the symptoms of fibromyalgia and its overlapping conditions, it is important to review treatment strategies that include those that would fall under the heading of *complementary*, *alternative*, or *integrative therapies*. These therapies include heath-care practices that are not considered part of conventional or mainstream Western medicine. Because fibromyalgia currently seems to be most effectively treated when multiple concurrent approaches are implemented, it is important to review treatment options beyond the pharmacological treatments discussed in Chapter 10.

def•i•ni•tion

According to the National Center for Complementary and Alternative Medicine ...

Complementary medicine is used together with conventional medicine. An example of a complementary therapy is using aromatherapy to help lessen a patient's discomfort following surgery.

Alternative medicine is used in place of conventional medicine. An example of an alternative therapy is using a special diet to treat cancer instead of undergoing surgery, radiation, or chemotherapy that has been recommended by a conventional doctor.

Integrative medicine is the practice of providing clinical services that treat the mind, body, and spirit.

It is not unusual to find a rheumatologist who is now practicing what is called integrative medicine, a mix of Western medicine along with complementary therapies in which there is evidence of safety and effectiveness. Unlike in the past, when an internist would only recommend approved conventional Western medicine, today it would not be unusual for an internist to recommend certain supplements or refer a patient for acupuncture treatments. In the search for more effective treatment options, traditional Western medicine is now researching therapies that have not been closely evaluated in the past.

In your development of an effective self-management plan, it is important that you carefully review and evaluate options that would be considered complementary or alternative therapies.

Acupuncture

Acupuncture originated in China some 3,500 years ago. It is one of the oldest systems of healing in the world and a main component of traditional Chinese medicine.

During a typical treatment for a chronic condition, 4 to 10 thin needles are placed into the skin at different points of the body. The thinking is that the insertion of the needles will help energy (*qi*) flow normally through the body. An acupuncture treatment usually consists of 6 to 12 treatments over a three-month period. Traditional acupuncturists might use additional therapies, including moxibustion (the burning of an herb just above the surface of the skin), massage, cupping, herbal preparations, exercises, and dietary modification.

 Fast Fact

Moxibustion is a traditional Chinese medicine technique that involves the burning of mugwort, a spongy herb, to facilitate healing. The purpose of moxibustion, as with most forms of traditional Chinese medicine, is to strengthen the blood, stimulate the flow of qi (or energy), and maintain general health.

The National Center for Complementary and Alternative Medicine, in Washington, D.C., believes that evidence from clinical research supports the use of acupuncture in treating pain conditions, especially migraine and tension headaches. Fibromyalgia researchers, however, have found variations in their research findings on whether it is effective in the treatment of fibromyalgia symptoms. Subjects in some studies experience a noticeable reduction in pain and other symptoms, while subjects in other studies have not reported much impact from acupuncture treatments. However, evidence seems to consistently indicate that acupuncture may be helpful in alleviating certain types of pain, decreasing gastrointestinal problems, and creating a relaxing experience for patients.

Massage

Therapeutic massage techniques involve the manipulation of the body's soft tissue (muscles, tendons, and ligaments) with the goal of helping to alleviate pain, stiffness, muscle spasm, and stress, and to promote relaxation and improved sleep. With the proper type of massage, you can feel physically and emotionally relaxed. Massage can help relax tight muscles, improve blood circulation, and increase the flow of oxygen and nutrients into the affected tissues. There are numerous types of therapeutic massage, which vary in intensity and suitability for people with fibromyalgia. These include Swedish, *deep tissue*, Shiatsu, acupressure, sports massage, Trager, reflexology, *myofascial release*, *trigger point therapy*, neuromuscular therapy, and medical massage. Some may be helpful to you and some may be too invasive or aggressive.

Fast Fact _____

Specialized forms of therapeutic massage that are often used to treat people with fibromyalgia and myofascial pain syndrome include the following:

Deep tissue. Releases the chronic patterns of tension in the body through slow strokes and deep finger pressure on the contracted areas, either following or going across the grain of muscles, tendons, and fascia. It is called deep tissue because it also focuses on the deeper layers of muscle tissue.

Myofascial release. Is a form of bodywork that is manipulative in nature and seeks to rebalance the body by releasing tension in the fascia. Long, stretching strokes are utilized to release muscular tension.

Trigger point therapy (also known as myotherapy or neuromuscular therapy). Applies concentrated finger pressure to "trigger points" (painful irritated areas in muscles) to break cycles of spasm and pain.

Just as you would with an exercise program, you should start your massage therapy slowly. Be sure the massage therapist is knowledgeable about fibromyalgia and is sensitive to your degree of pain sensitivity. Before making an appointment for a massage, you may want to find out how often the therapist has treated people with fibromyalgia or other chronic pain conditions. It is difficult at best to recommend a particular type of massage because people with fibromyalgia tend to like different intensities of pressure in massage therapy. I personally cannot tolerate any type of deep tissue massage, but I know people with fibromyalgia who believe that this is the only type of treatment that can help release their tight, sore muscles.

The massage therapist should ask you questions about your general health and why you have decided to have a massage. Do not be afraid to ask for credentials and whether he or she is a member of the American Massage Therapy Association (AMTA) (www.amtamassage.org). Thirty-three states have now passed legislation to regulate massage therapy. The primary national credential is *Nationally Certified in Therapeutic Massage and Bodywork*, which is designated by the initials NCTMB. The designation NCTMB is awarded by the National Certification Board for Therapeutic Massage and Bodywork (NCBTMB), which is a nonprofit corporation. Education is another criterion upon which you can evaluate massage therapists. AMTA recommends you look for a graduate of a training program that has been accredited by the Commission on Massage Therapy Accreditation (COMTA) or an agency with equivalent standards.

Chiropractic Manipulation

Chiropractic treatment, which utilizes joint manipulation, has been in use since the late nineteenth century. The belief was that poor spine alignment caused various disorders, and they could be corrected by skillful hands-on manual manipulation. Along with spinal manipulation, most chiropractors also use soft tissue massage, stretching, and hot and cold therapy. At this time there is limited research on the use of chiropractic manipulation to treat people with fibromyalgia. It appears that it is most helpful as a form of stretching. To find a qualified chiropractor, talk to your health-care professional or contact the American Chiropractic Association (www.amerchiro.org).

Healthy Alternative

The application of heat or cold is a common type of passive, noninvasive, and non-addictive pain therapy.

Heat can be applied to the painful area of the body by way of a hot/moist compress, a dry or moist heating pad, hydrotherapy or hot water pool, or commercial chemical/gel packs. Heat therapy draws blood into the target tissues. The increased blood flow provides needed oxygen and nutrients and removes cell wastes. The warmth decreases muscle spasms, relaxes tense muscles, relieves pain, and can increase range of motion.

Cold can be applied in the form of commercial cold packs, ice cubes, or iced towels/compresses. Even a bag of frozen peas can make a great cold compress. Cold therapy slows circulation, which reduces inflammation, muscle spasms, and pain.

The application of hot and cold compresses can be done independently or in combination with one another. Ask your health-care professional which might work best for you.

Physical Therapy (PT)

According to Stephanie Bolling, M.S., P.T., O.C.S., founder of the Los Angeles area–based Arthritis Therapy Specialists, the goal of physical therapy is to help restore function, improve mobility and independence, relieve pain, and prevent or limit permanent physical disabilities for people dealing with musculoskeletal conditions. Individuals who seek help from a physical therapist should be sure that the therapist specializes in the treatment of rheumatological conditions. The physical therapist should understand the symptom components of fibromyalgia and implement a program specifically designed to help decrease the symptoms of fibromyalgia. A knowledgeable specialist will empower you by teaching you specific exercises and stretches that should be performed when different muscle flare-ups occur.

Ms. Bolling explains that a physical therapy evaluation for fibromyalgia should assess the following:

- Muscle spasms and most tender points
- Muscle flexibility and strength
- Posture analysis
- Body mechanics
- Gait analysis
- Functional limitations
- Aerobic activity
- Fatigue
- Sleep hygiene
- Stress or anxiety level
- Patient's goals

A proper physical therapy treatment should consist of the following:

- Manual therapy consisting of joint and soft tissue mobilization, manipulation, or massage to decrease muscle spasms or tender points (manual therapy might not be tolerated due to hypersensitivity)
- Individualized stretching program
- Proper posture training

- ◆ Body mechanics training

- ◆ Breathing and stress reduction training

- ◆ Proper sleep hygiene training

- ◆ Proper aerobic activity training

- ◆ Safe, individualized strength training (Pilates recommended)

- ◆ Functional activity training

- ◆ Self-management home treatments to reduce pain during flare-ups

- ◆ Communication with doctors regarding patient care

Fast Fact _____

No matter what activity or therapy is recommended to you, it is imperative that you listen to your body. Do not participate in any activity that is too intense for you to perform or which leaves you in more pain than you can tolerate. It is always recommended that you start slowly and then gradually try more intense types of treatments. Remember that what works for one person may not work for another.

Aquatic Therapy

Aquatic therapy is an effective exercise option for many people with fibromyalgia. In a pool, you can perform aerobic exercises without the weight-bearing and joint compression of land-based exercises. The water allows you to be buoyant, which can give the freedom of movement that pain might have taken away from you. As you're immersed in a warm-water pool (heated between 91°F and 94°F), your muscles and mind can relax without effort.

As you slowly increase your stamina in the pool, you can achieve a greater level of overall physical fitness. Aquatic therapy helps build endurance and increases arm and leg strength, flexibility, and balance. It allows you to improve or maintain your ability to walk, climb stairs, and participate in other types of exercise and

Healthy Alternative
Most YMCAs nationwide offer a program that was developed by the Arthritis Foundation called Twinges in the Hinges. It is a gentle aquatic exercise program that takes place in a heated pool and provides for full body range of motion. Participating in this program is an excellent way to reintroduce movement into your life.

athletic activities. Group aquatic classes also give you an opportunity to socialize and participate. Watsu is a therapy that combines stretching with water therapy.

Occupational Therapy (OT)

The occupational therapist's goal is to help individuals who have developed health conditions that affect their independence and ability to perform daily activities. As a trained and licensed health-care professional, the OT can evaluate the impact that fibromyalgia has on you and help you lessen or overcome your limitations at home or work. The OT works cooperatively with the other members of the health-care team to customize a treatment program that will give you ways to better manage your active life. An OT can also offer guidance to family members to help them understand the recommendations and creative solutions that have been made to improve your daily functionality. Often physical therapists will work with an OT to assist with exercise and other therapies that help improve physical balance, strength, and flexibility.

Therapy for the Body and Mind

Other forms of physical movement including yoga, Tai Chi, Pilates, and Feldenkrais can integrate the mind/body experience into exercise. Instead of focusing on the hard, fast, and intense movements of other forms of exercise, these practices allow you to increase your strength and balance through visualization, meditation, and slow, precise stretching. Each of these techniques affects the participant in different ways. Always start slowly and check the qualifications of the teacher before you experiment with any kind of mind/body exercise program.

Yoga

The practice of yoga began more than 6,000 years ago to help individuals experience spiritual enlightenment. The postures of yoga were developed to help balance the body, feelings, and thoughts in order to give practitioners an overall greater awareness and feeling of peace. Today, yoga is seen as a way to keep a positive focus and help ensure overall physical and mental well-being. Hatha yoga is the most widely practiced yoga in the United States. In this type of practice the focus is on postures (asanas), breathing exercises (pranayama), and guided relaxation. Hatha yoga is part of classical yoga (raja yoga—the royal path).

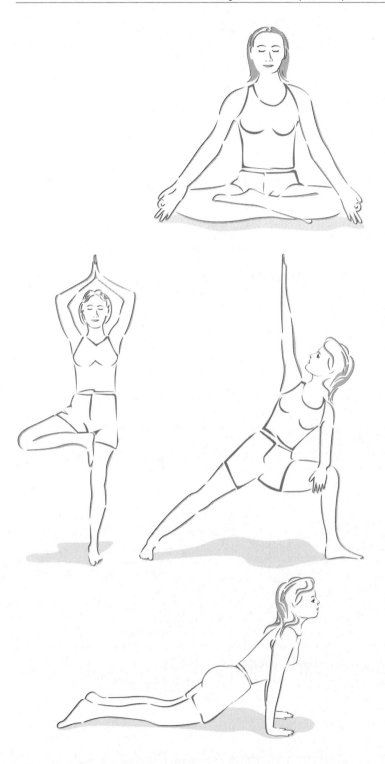

Yoga positions, or asanas, are excellent exercises for stretching, toning muscles, and massaging the body. Yoga postures bring physical as well as mental stability to your health. Yoga positions were developed thousands of years ago and have evolved over the centuries. They exercise the nerves, glands, ligaments, and muscles of the body.

(Illustration courtesy of Craig Kennedy.)

Yoga positions can be done while sitting, standing, or lying down. The examples shown here are popular yoga poses; however, less strenuous positions can also provide health benefits.

(Illustrations courtesy of Craig Kennedy.)

Pain Signal _____

Because yoga has been practiced for thousands of years, there are many different forms and different philosophies as to how yoga should be taught. There are also a variety of certification programs, none of which is touted as better than another. As you begin exploring yoga classes in your community, it is important to chat with the teacher and be sure that the teacher and type of yoga that is being taught fits your needs. Be sure to ask the following questions:

- Is the yoga being taught vigorous or gentle?
- Is there a beginner's class or one for people who have health problems?
- How long has the teacher been teaching?
- Can I participate at my own level if the class goes beyond my capabilities?

Picture This/Lessons Learned

Picture This:

After spending months and then years in bed because of fibromyalgia, I didn't know how to find a way to become active again. I called my local hospital and was told about a yoga school that had been in our community for more than 25 years. When I called the center, I was given the name of an instructor who did in-home yoga classes. Ila, who became my teacher and friend, played a huge role in helping me learn the techniques of relaxation that eventually would be instrumental in helping me learn how to deal with my pain. My yoga classes took place on my living room floor. For months I just laid on my yoga mat doing deep relaxation exercises and learning how to relax my mind and body. As time progressed I learned how to do yoga postures, breathing exercises, and meditation that strengthened and helped balance my mind and body.

Lessons Learned:

There are people in your community who can help you along your path to better health. Be open to new ideas and look to those in your wellness community who might be able to guide or assist you with classes or people who can provide you with new alternatives for better health care.

Tai Chi

Tai Chi was originally developed thousands of years ago in China as a martial art, but has been redefined as a way to reconnect the mind and body. Tai Chi has been described as "meditation in movement," which will help you to achieve "joy in the movement." The premise is to keep your feet on the ground, with a relaxed "puppet-like" attitude, supporting a straight spine while your movements "follow your breath" and your mind stays still.

Through your movement, you are aligning your body to enhance the flow of energy. As you dance or begin to move, you become aware that your feet are grounded and that your eyes are aware but not focused. By practicing Tai Chi you are practicing being "in the now," yet being aware of everything around you. Those who practice Tai Chi explain that it is not about trying, but rather about letting go. For people with fibromyalgia, practicing Tai Chi can help them understand that they don't have to struggle, but rather can learn to let go and not resist. The advantage of this form of exercise is that there is no right way to do it. Even without physically moving, you can visualize your movements and achieve mental benefit.

Pilates

Unlike yoga and Tai Chi, Pilates was developed in the early twentieth century. The Pilates method is not just a set of exercises performed with Pilates equipment, but a complete approach to developing body awareness. It is a conditioning program that is meant to focus on subtle movements to improve muscle control and flexibility, coordination, balance, tone, and strength. Pilates utilizes proper breathing techniques and is very dependent on a trusting relationship between you and the Pilates teacher. By applying the Pilates technique of slow, precise movements, the goal is to strengthen and stretch the body's core muscles.

Pain Signal

As you begin exploring different types of complementary therapies, you will realize how important it is to check out the credentials of those who teach the various types of classes. When looking for a Pilates instructor, don't be afraid to ask a lot of questions. For example …

- ◆ Can I visit your Pilates studio?
- ◆ Do you (the Pilates teacher) clean the equipment after each student?
- ◆ Are students left unattended?
- ◆ Can I observe you teaching your students?
- ◆ Can you provide me with student references?
- ◆ Do you work with students who have fibromyalgia?

Reiki

The name Reiki is made up of two words: Rei, which means "God's Wisdom or the Higher Power," and Ki, which is "life force energy." So Reiki is actually "spiritually guided life force energy."

The practice of Reiki originated in Japan and is based on the belief that when a person's spiritual energy is channeled through a trained Reiki practitioner, their spirit can be healed, which in turn causes the physical body to be healed. Reiki is a simple, natural, and safe method of spiritual healing and self-improvement that is now practiced around the world.

Feldenkrais

Like Pilates, the Feldenkrais Method was developed in the early twentieth century. It focuses on the connection between movement and thought. Practitioners learn to focus on the way they move so that they can increase ease and range of motion and improve flexibility and coordination. They discover their movement habits, and develop new ways of movement. Like the therapies discussed previously, Feldenkrais focuses on the physical—but also offers practitioners a "relaxation response" that may make them feel more balanced and at peace.

Supplements

Supplements are vitamins and minerals taken in pill form to supplement what you ingest in the foods you eat. There is research that supports the fact that people with fibromyalgia often have low or below-normal levels of magnesium, B-12, vitamin D, and zinc.

Although many health-care professionals believe that proper nutrition can be achieved through proper eating habits, there is a school of thought that believes that supplementation is another effective way of ensuring that your body is receiving the vitamins and minerals necessary for proper nutritional health. There are many different types of vitamins, and each of them has its own specific benefit to various parts and functions of the body. Some vitamins help ward off disease, while others help build strong bones and muscles. Even the *Journal of the American Medical Association* recommends that everyone—regardless of age and health status—take a daily multivitamin.

Fast Fact

In the 1994 *Dietary Supplement Health and Education Act (DSHEA)*, a dietary supplement is defined as a product that might include vitamins, minerals, herbs or other botanicals, amino acids, and substances such as enzymes, organ tissues, and metabolites. These products can come in many forms, including tablets, capsules, gel caps, liquids, powders, extracts, and concentrates. Under the DSHEA, dietary supplements are considered foods, not drugs.

Registered *nutritionists* are primarily concerned with the prevention and treatment of illnesses through proper dietary care. They evaluate the diets of clients suffering from medical disorders and suggest ways of fighting various health problems by modifying the intake of certain foods. They advise individuals and groups on the nutritional practices that will promote good health. In some cases they might advise their patients that they would benefit from nutritional therapy or supplementation.

def•i•ni•tion

The Certification Board for Nutrition Specialists defines a **nutritionist** as "a health specialist who devotes his or her professional activity exclusively to food/nutrition science, preventative nutrition, diseases related to nutrient deficiencies, and the use of nutrient manipulation to enhance the clinical response to human diseases."

Herbs

Herbal remedies are medicinal preparations derived from plants. It is very important to remember that even though they are natural substances, they cannot be used haphazardly. Herbs can be strong medicine and can cause adverse reactions. Before trying any herbal remedy, be sure that you are familiar with what it does, how it is used, and any possible side effects it can cause. Never exceed the recommended dose.

A doctor should monitor the use of any medicinal herb, making sure it does not produce a dangerous interaction with medications already prescribed. Also, if a sensitivity or allergic reaction occurs, consult a health-care professional immediately. If you are aware of the risks and are willing to do some research (check the Herbs Research Foundation at www.herbs.org), you may benefit from herbs, especially in the treatment of nausea, sleeplessness, anxiety, poor circulation, memory loss, constipation, and fatigue.

Electromagnetic Therapy

Electromagnetic fields (EMFs) are invisible lines of force that surround all electrical devices. Electromagnetic therapy is a recently developed complementary therapy, which exposes a patient to varying intensities and frequencies of electromagnetic impulses. According to William Pawluk, M.D., assistant professor, Johns Hopkins University School of Medicine, "Indirect benefits of magnetic fields on physiologic function are on: circulation, muscle, edema, tissue oxygen, inflammation, healing, prostaglandins, cellular metabolism, and cell energy levels."

Alternative Medical Thought

Alternative medicine is not as "alternative" as it has been in the past. Conventional Western medicine still remains the traditional focus of medical practice in the United States, while other forms of medical thought are not as often seen as outlandish or unacceptable as previously considered. No longer do all physicians reject anything other than "science-based" methods or medicine that falls under biomedical terms. For example, acupuncture is now often accepted as a complementary therapy, rather than an alternative therapy.

Naturopathic medicine and homeopathic medicine have recently become more popular. Once thought of as alternative, they are now sometimes considered to be complementary options.

Naturopathic Medicine

Naturopathic medicine is a natural approach to healing that takes into consideration the integrity of the whole person. The belief is that the body has the ability to maintain and restore health, and it is the physician's role to facilitate this process, helping to remove obstacles of poor health and disease and to support a healthy internal and external environment. Naturopathic physicians help determine the underlying cause(s) of illness that are expressed as symptoms. The causes may be on the physical, mental, emotional, or spiritual level, and the physician will treat the cause rather than suppressing the symptom.

Homeopathic Medicine

Homeopathic medicine is an alternative medical system. In homeopathic medicine, the belief is that "like cures like." The concept behind homeopathic medicine is that a cure will result when small amounts of a substance, which are normally given at a higher or more concentrated dose, would actually cause those symptoms. A homeopath will provide his or her patients with small, highly diluted quantities of medicinal substances to cure symptoms.

Your Notes and Questions on Complementary, Alternative, and Integrative Therapies

Now that you have read an overview of some of the complementary and alternative treatment options for people with fibromyalgia, make notes on areas that you are interested in and think about questions for your health-care professional.

When faced with illnesses such as fibromyalgia, which have proven difficult to treat strictly by traditional medicine, health-care professionals and patients alike have turned to complementary methods of treatment. The problem is in knowing which options are viable if you don't have clinical studies on which to base your decisions. Just remember that when evaluating complementary or alternative options, you should always be aware of the following:

- Claims that seem too good to be true

- Treatments that are overly expensive

- Practices that feel wrong to your *instincts*

- Something your health-care professional has warned you against

def•i•ni•tion _____

The term **instinct** refers to feelings and drives that are not learned, but rather come from innate animal behavior, which results in such natural practices as nursing or caring for your young. When you are advised to pay attention to your instincts, you are being asked to base your actions on your internal feelings, rather than a response that has been taught to you.

The Least You Need to Know

- It is important to review treatment strategies, including those that would fall under the heading "complementary, alternative, or integrative therapies."

- Integrative medicine is a mix of Western medicine and complementary therapies in which there is evidence of safety and effectiveness.

- ◆ Complementary medicine is a type of therapy (for example, aromatherapy, massage, and supplements) that is used together with conventional Western medicine.

- ◆ Alternative medicine is used in place of conventional medicine.

- ◆ No longer do all physicians reject anything other than science-based methods or medicine that falls under biomedical terms.

- ◆ When faced with illnesses such as fibromyalgia (which has proven difficult to treat strictly by traditional medicine), health-care professionals and patients alike have turned to alternative methods of treatment.

Chapter 12

Behavioral Interventions

In This Chapter

- ◆ Seeking counseling and emotional support
- ◆ Benefiting from the long-lasting pain relief of CBT
- ◆ Improving your health through biofeedback
- ◆ Benefiting from informal support-group meetings
- ◆ Using art and music as ways to help with fibromyalgia symptoms

For years, people with fibromyalgia have been fighting the notion that fibromyalgia is a psychological or mental illness. Because there have only been limited treatment options available to people with fibromyalgia, the emphasis has been on learning how to "deal with the pain." Today we know that fibromyalgia is not a psychological illness, and we recognize the need for future treatment options to *treat* symptoms, rather than just teach the patient how to live with them. We must recognize, though, that behavioral modification interventions, which involve techniques and strategies that change behavior, can have a positive impact as part of the overall treatment plan.

Everyone who has a chronic illness must deal with both the physical symptoms and the emotional toll of the illness. When dealing with fibromyalgia, you need to identify and explore treatment modalities that provide physiological as well as psychological help. The goal is to increase your chances for an improved outcome. By implementing behavioral interventions along with other types of treatment modalities, you can increase your chances of improving both your physical and emotional health.

It is important that you don't let your fears or prejudices keep you from taking advantage of all the treatment options available to you. If you think that counseling is only for people who are weak, or that cognitive behavioral therapy is only for someone who is crazy, then you will be limiting your treatment options. Remember that it is always important to treat the whole person, which includes the body, mind, and spirit. This chapter teaches you about a variety of behavioral interventions that just might be beneficial to you!

Seeking Emotional Counseling

It is not surprising that people with a chronic pain illness may develop secondary psychological complaints such as depression, fear, anger, and anxiety. Fibromyalgia is *not* a psychological illness; however, all physiological illnesses also affect you emotionally. It's important to remember that each person is a complete entity: body, mind, and spirit.

Because our physical experiences are intertwined with our emotional experiences (and vice versa), it is not difficult to understand that it is beneficial to seek treatment for your physical and your emotional self. Certain things that can be part of the fibromyalgia experience can cause you to become frustrated and even depressed. For example, experiencing a prolonged pre-diagnosis period, poor or limited support from the medical community, lack of understanding from family members and friends, severe chronic pain and fatigue that can last for weeks and even months at a time, changes that disrupt your lifestyle, and the inability to do the things that you used to do—all these experiences affect your emotional health. Even the most optimistic person can become emotionally challenged when faced with the symptoms and life-altering challenges that can result from fibromyalgia.

Although admitting that you are unhappy or even depressed might be a new and difficult experience for you, it is important to remember that these feelings are not a sign of weakness. Asking for emotional support or seeking out psychological treatment(s) can be an important aspect of your overall health improvement.

Fast Fact _____

People with good emotional health can keep problems in perspective and have learned ways to cope with stress and negative issues. There are times, however, when people who have always had good emotional health can have emotional problems or even suffer from mental illnesses such as depression and anxiety. During these times they feel out of control of their thoughts, feelings, and behaviors. That's when they need to seek help from a doctor or a counselor.

Psychological and physiological symptoms can be treated with pharmacological agents or through behavioral interventions. Robert Bennett, M.D., believes that psychological counseling, particularly the use of techniques such as cognitive restructuring and biofeedback, may benefit some individuals who are having difficulties coping with the realities of living with their physical pain and associated psychological symptoms.

Developing these symptoms isn't something you should feel guilty or embarrassed about. Learning to adjust to new challenges and circumstances can cause anyone to need emotional support. If you made the decision to start a new career, it would not be unusual to seek out counseling or get assistance from an expert in the field. In dealing with lifestyle changes and emotional issues, it also makes sense to seek out counseling or expert assistance!

Along with the various types of medical treatments that treat the physical aspects of fibromyalgia, there are treatment options that can treat the mental, emotional, and spiritual aspects of your health. The following sections look at the options for treating mental and emotional aspects of the disease.

Fast Fact _____

Depression is not an emotional weakness or something that you can just will away. Rather, it is a complicated medical condition caused by chemical imbalances in the brain.

Cognitive Behavioral Therapy (CBT)

Cognitive behavioral therapy (CBT) has been well studied as an *additive* approach to the traditional medical treatment of chronic pain and fibromyalgia. As David Williams, Ph.D., of the University of Michigan, points out, if two individuals have fibromyalgia, their reactions to pain will differ. Your own individual coping skills, learned behaviors, and emotional reactions will influence not only how you will react to pain, but how you will experience it.

CBT can help you learn how to manage the symptoms of worsening pain. By learning to recognize your maladaptive thoughts and practice specific techniques for pain management, you may produce improvements in your overall pain. The major philosophical assumption of CBT is that by changing your thinking and your belief system, you in turn change your behavior. This in no way means that you have to "think yourself well." If, however, you accept the fact that there is a strong connection between what you think and how you feel emotionally *and* physically, you will benefit by learning how to develop skills to help change your thinking and develop an aptitude to solve problems.

Picture This/Lessons Learned

Picture This:

When I first became ill with fibromyalgia, it was very easy for me to constantly focus on my pain. I would continuously report to my husband (or whoever was with me) where it hurt and how much it hurt. My health-care professional told me to stop thinking so much about the pain. This just infuriated me, because I felt like it was an unreasonable request. One day my husband asked me to try to think about something else. I tried to explain to him that, "...asking me to stop thinking about my pain is like asking me not to think of a purple elephant!" The minute you say, "Don't think of a purple elephant," that is the first thing that comes to your mind. His comment to me was, "...but once you have thought of the purple elephant, then it starts to fade from your mind—you don't just keep thinking 'purple elephant, purple elephant', over and over again! You want to stop thinking about that elephant and start to think about something else." It was with that comment I realized that I needed to recognize that my pain (the purple elephant) was going to come into my thoughts, but that I could learn how to fade it out of my thoughts as I focused on other things.

Lessons Learned:

Oftentimes I am asked if I still have pain. Though I have developed a self-management plan that has reduced my pain tremendously, I do still have to deal with pain. However, just like the purple elephant, I don't think about it very often. I have learned to put it in the back of my thoughts, where it can't control or take over my life. You have a choice: focus on the pain, or don't focus on the pain.

Dr. Williams explains that CBT usually includes three phases:

◆ Educational phase. Learning about your illness and your role in pain management.

◆ Skills–training phase. Training in cognitive and behavioral pain-coping skills, such as relaxation, pleasant activity scheduling, problem-solving, and sleep hygiene.

◆ Application phase. Learning to apply your skills in real-life situations.

Learning to implement the skills of CBT will take time and practice. Although you might not immediately appreciate the benefits of CBT, once you do experience them, the benefits may last longer than those of other types of treatment.

Biofeedback

Biofeedback is a treatment technique in which people are trained to improve their own health by using signals from the body. A person is hooked up to one of numerous types of biofeedback machines. The machine can detect sensitive internal bodily functions (such as heart rate) and report (through lights, bells, graphs, pictures, and so on) important information that will help both the patient and therapist gauge and direct the progress of treatment.

For patients, the biofeedback machine acts as a sixth sense that allows them to visually recognize the activities going on inside their bodies. It can also act as a reward system for patients, letting them know (through lights, bells, and pictures) when they are mentally changing the responses happening in their bodies. For example, the machine can pick up electrical signals in muscles and then report this activity back to patients in the form of a bright flashing light, or a line on a screen that moves upward with tension and downward with muscle relaxation. The light flashes faster or the line moves upward if the machine picks up signals that reflect tension in muscles. With this information, patients can recognize what is happening in their bodies and make an active mental attempt to change those responses.

The biofeedback process has shown that people have more control over their involuntary bodily functions (heart rate, digestion, pain, etc.) than once thought. But nature limits the extent of such control. Biofeedback puts a lot of demands on patients, requiring them to practice biofeedback techniques every day. The lessons learned, however, may help patients feel more in control over migraine and tension headaches, muscle tension and pain, high and low blood pressure, digestive problems, and blood circulation.

Biofeedback therapists also use relaxation tapes and exercises to help individuals learn how to relax their minds and bodies. Specialists who provide biofeedback training range from psychiatrists and psychologists to dentists, internists, nurses, and physical therapists. To find a biofeedback therapist, ask your health-care professional, state biofeedback society, the Association for Applied Psychophysiology and Biofeedback (www.aapb.org), or the psychology department at your local university.

Picture This/Lessons Learned

Picture This:

I never realized how important it is to pay attention to the signals that your body gives you. There was a time when, month after month, I suffered from migraine headaches that felt like I had been shot through the head with a high-powered gun. Although there was a series of warning signals that preceded the migraines, I was so out of touch with my body that I never recognized them. After several sessions of sitting in front of a biofeedback machine, which showed me a graphic illustration when my body was becoming tense, my breathing was becoming rapid, and my pulse was increasing, I learned how to "listen" to my body. After I recognized the signals of a migraine coming on, I could then practice relaxation techniques that often helped to decrease the intensity of the migraine or even prevented it completely.

Lessons Learned:

It is easy to depend on medication to help reduce pain, prevent anxiety, or even help you sleep. But by learning how to listen to my body and control some of its reactions through my thoughts, I found that I could reduce the amount of medication I had to take. There are times when medications are necessary, but it is exciting to learn that there are times when I can become more aware of my body's signals and, through various techniques, affect my body's reactions through thought.

Individual Therapy

Individual therapy consists of one-on-one counseling where the client spends individual time with the primary therapist, medical provider, or specialty therapists. Such a working relationship may last for only a few sessions or may continue for much longer, depending on your needs. Although talking to a counselor for the first time can feel awkward or embarrassing, individual therapy can be effective in helping you deal with a variety of issues and help improve your quality of life.

Supportive Group Therapy

Group therapy is the process in which individuals with similar issues or health conditions meet in a group setting with a designated leader (facilitator, therapist, or heath-care professional) to benefit from an exchange of experiences and thoughts, and to discuss positive ways to solve problems. It is the responsibility of the group's leader to keep the dynamics and direction of the group in line with the goals of the session.

People with fibromyalgia may benefit from both structured group-therapy sessions and more informal support-group meetings. In a medically directed forum, participants usually are the ones who decide the topics to be discussed and the direction of the discussion (with the guidance of the health-care professional). In a support-group meeting, an expert usually shares information that is then discussed, questioned, and absorbed.

It is important to be aware of the goals of the group. It is not helpful to be a part of a negative, self-serving group that is not focused on learning ways to better your situation. Be aware of groups that focus on one person, or one in which everyone is complaining rather than focusing on sharing techniques to help resolve your health challenges.

A support-group meeting should fill the following needs:

- ◆ Provide social interaction
- ◆ Offer personal support
- ◆ Be an informational exchange
- ◆ Promote physical and emotional healing
- ◆ Provide techniques for dealing with problematic issues
- ◆ Give individuals a safe place where they are not being judged or criticized

Healthy Alternative

If you find yourself attending a support group where the focus is on whining and complaining, you need to remove yourself from the group immediately. Negative exchanges can only have a negative effect on your health. Support groups are supposed to be supportive, healthy exchanges of positive and helpful information that will move you forward in your development of a self-management plan. Many good support groups will have an expert speaker or informative handouts as part of the meeting's program.

One of the most important aspects of a support group is that it can offer you a place where you are surrounded by people who understand what you are going through. A support group should be a place where you don't feel like you are being judged. Living with a chronic illness can often make you feel alone and insecure. By joining a support group where you feel accepted, your overall self-confidence will improve and you will become less likely to feel isolated and afraid.

Art and Music Therapy

The concept that art and music have healing and life-enhancing capabilities is not a new one. Through the process of appreciating or creating various forms of art and music, you may be able to improve your ability to deal with pain and stress. Art and music can shift your focus from the negative things you are experiencing to pleasure and self-expression. You may find that this will help you to cope, heal, and enhance your life.

You can use art and music on your own as a way to help you with your fibromyalgia symptoms, or you can work with music or art therapists. Both types of therapists hold Master's degrees in their fields and work in clinical settings, community facilities, schools and universities, and private practices. The goal is to create—through whatever form the therapy takes—in order to facilitate positive changes in behavior and emotional well-being.

Hypnosis

Through hypnosis, a person with fibromyalgia can be given the suggestion to exercise more, to sleep better, and even to have a decreased sensitivity to pain. As a complementary therapy to traditional medicine, hypnosis puts you in a trancelike state that opens you to suggestion. When in a hypnotic state, you feel completely relaxed and can focus intensely on the subject at hand. Each individual has his or her own level of susceptibility to hypnosis, which will determine the level of success you will experience with this form of therapy.

It is important that you work with a well-trained, trustworthy hypnotherapist who develops realistic goals. While in the hypnotic trance, the therapist can suggest changes in behaviors, thoughts, and feelings. If these suggestions meet your needs, you will be able to reinforce the suggestions at a later time. To ensure that you are working with a trained professional, ask for a referral from your health-care professional or from your local hospital or university.

Although hypnosis has been criticized because of its use as entertainment in stage shows, it is being reevaluated as a useful therapy. David Spiegel, M.D., of Stanford University, believes that hypnosis is a psychological state in which changes in brain function occur. With additional research, the role of hypnosis in the treatment of chronic pain may be better understood and more often utilized.

> **Healthy Alternative**
>
> If you feel like you *are* fibromyalgia rather than a person, it is important to remind yourself that you still have the same heart and soul as you did before you got fibromyalgia. You are not your illness! You are an individual who is just as valuable as anyone else.

Faith

Although faith is not a behavioral intervention, it is a practice that can have an incredible impact on how you feel. Some individuals feel that their faith is an integral part of their healing.

A 1995 study at Dartmouth College in Hanover, New Hampshire, monitored 250 people after open-heart surgery and concluded that those who had religious connections were 12 times less likely to die than those who had none.

Duke University researchers assessed 1,000 hospital patients from 1987 to 1989 and found that patients who drew on their religious practices, including prayer, coped far better than those who didn't.

For many people, scientific studies are not necessary to prove the power of faith. Many people with fibromyalgia have found that the counsel of clergy or the practice of prayer is beneficial to the health of their mind, body, and soul.

Your Notes and Questions on Behavioral Interventions

Now that you have read an overview of some behavioral interventions for people with fibromyalgia, make notes on areas that you are interested in and develop questions for your health-care professional.

The Least You Need to Know

- ◆ Learning to adjust to new challenges and circumstances can cause anyone to need emotional support.
- ◆ Fibromyalgia is not a psychological illness, but all physiological illnesses also have an emotional component.

◆ By learning to recognize your maladaptive thoughts and practicing specific techniques for pain management, you will likely produce improvements in your overall pain.

◆ Training in cognitive and behavioral pain-coping skills can help with relaxation, problem solving, and sleep hygiene.

◆ Shifting your focus from the negative things that you are experiencing and onto pleasure and self-expression may offer you a way to cope, heal, and enhance your life.

◆ Although faith is not a behavioral intervention, it is a practice that can have an incredible impact on how you feel.

Chapter 13

Treating Overlapping Conditions

In This Chapter

- ◆ Treating and assessing overlapping conditions
- ◆ Treating sleep disorders
- ◆ Understanding irritable bowel syndrome
- ◆ Defining fibro fog
- ◆ Treating migraine headaches in multiple ways
- ◆ Treating restless legs syndrome

As you learned in Chapter 1, it is not unusual for a person with fibromyalgia to experience a large variety of symptoms other than pain. Many of these symptoms might not be specifically related to fibromyalgia, but rather might indicate the presence of other chronic and acute conditions that are frequently seen in people with fibromyalgia. Sometimes, the treatments for these conditions are easier and more effective than the options for treating specific fibromyalgia symptoms. This chapter covers the most prevalent overlapping conditions and suggests ways to manage their symptoms effectively.

Assessing Overlapping Conditions

Overlapping conditions are a case of bad news and good news. The bad news is that people with fibromyalgia experience a variety of overlapping conditions; the good news is that many options are available to successfully treat these conditions. If you can get relief from the symptoms of the overlapping conditions (such as headaches, migraines, irritable bowel syndrome, restless legs syndrome, and so on), your fibromyalgia pain and fatigue will often become less pronounced as well.

As you and your health-care professional work toward relieving the symptoms and discomfort of these other conditions, it will have a positive effect on your overall health. For example, treating and getting your migraine headaches under control or finding the right medications to relieve your restless legs syndrome will reduce the number of symptoms you are dealing with and alleviate some of your physical and emotional distress. Focusing on the overlapping conditions that you have been diagnosed with is a good place to start your quest to become healthier.

Healthy Alternative

When you first take note of all your medical complaints, ask your health-care professional which are the easiest to treat. The answer may not be the most concerning or distressful of your complaints, but if you eliminate at least some of your concerns, the challenges in front of you won't seem so overwhelming. Also, as you see progress in these areas, it will help you feel more positive about a good future outcome in other areas!

Sleep Disorders

When you experience the sleep disorders that can accompany fibromyalgia, it's hard to believe that you ever took sleep for granted. Not only is the inability to get a good night's sleep frustrating, it also has a major impact on overall health. Good sleep is necessary to produce certain essential hormones and chemicals that help regenerate certain parts of the body, especially in the brain.

Researchers believe that the primary function of sleep might very well be cerebral restoration. After an individual experiences even short periods of insomnia or restless sleep, certain neurochemicals can begin to malfunction, visibly affecting a person's behavior and preventing them from functioning at their full potential. It is known that a person experiences changes in glucose tolerance and endocrine function simply by not getting enough deep, restorative sleep. The muscles of the body are not able to regenerate unless the deep stages of sleep are reached.

Fast Fact _____

When we are awake and resting, our brains generate "alpha" waves at a frequency of 8 to 13 per second. When we are in deep sleep, our brains begin to generate slower "delta" waves at a rate of less than 3.5 per second. Many people with fibromyalgia have a disordered pattern of brain activity during sleep called "alpha-delta sleep" in which alpha (arousal) waves occur during stages of deep sleep when only delta waves should be present. By being jolted back to lighter sleep, they are unable to get the benefits of deeper sleep stages such as muscle repair, which depends on growth hormone secretion during deep sleep. This lack of sleep accentuates the fatigue and musculoskeletal pain that most people with fibromyalgia experience.

It is vital to diagnose specific sleep disorders when present, such as sleep apnea and restless legs syndrome, so that proper medical treatment can be implemented. (To learn more about specific types of sleep disorders, go to Chapter 15.) The symptom of nonrestorative sleep is central to fibromyalgia; however, the treatment can be different for each individual based on what is causing the lack of sleep.

Fast Fact _____

The following are some of the most common types of sleep disorders experienced by people with fibromyalgia:

Insomnia is poor-quality sleep, including the inability to fall asleep, stay asleep, or wake up feeling refreshed.

Sleep apnea is a sleep disorder in which a person stops breathing throughout the night for periods of up to two minutes. It is usually accompanied by loud snoring. These periods of breathing stoppages disrupt sleep cycles and deprive the body of needed oxygen. Restless legs syndrome (RLS) is a disorder causing unpleasant crawling or tingling sensations in the legs and feet that causes you to feel like you must get up and move to find relief. Narcolepsy is somewhat rare in people with fibromyalgia, but those who have it experience frequent "sleep attacks" at various times of the day. These are attacks in which the individual falls asleep at inappropriate times that can last from several seconds to more than 30 minutes.

Nonrestorative sleep refers to the feeling of being unrefreshed or tired following adequate sleep time. This kind of sleep disorder is common in people with depression, chronic fatigue syndrome, and periodic limb movement disorder.

There are many effective management tools that can be used to help treat sleep disorders, including …

◆ Exercise.

◆ Addressing psychological problems, such as depression and anxiety.

◆ The use of medications, such as certain antidepressants, benzodiazepines, antispasmodics, and muscle relaxants.

◆ In cases of sleep apnea, the use of dental appliances, a *CPAP (Continuous Positive Airway Pressure) machine,* or surgery.

def•i•ni•tion

A **CPAP machine** (or Continuous Positive Airway Pressure machine) provides therapy for those who suffer with obstructive sleep apnea. A flexible tube connects the machine with a mask that is worn over the nose and/or mouth. The CPAP works by pushing air through the airway passage at a pressure high enough to prevent apneas, which are caused by obstruction of the breathing passage. The pressure is adjusted depending on the level of the patient's sleep apnea.

◆ Relaxation exercises.

◆ Creating a sleep-conducive environment.

◆ Adjusting your diet to aid digestion and avoiding stimulants like alcohol, sugar, and caffeine.

Irritable Bowel Syndrome

Irritable bowel syndrome (IBS) is a functional GI disorder characterized by abdominal pain and altered bowel habits in the absence of any organic pathology findings. The symptoms of IBS include cramping, bloating, abdominal pain, constipation, diarrhea, or alternating constipation and diarrhea. Between 50 and 75 percent of people with fibromyalgia may be diagnosed with IBS. The symptoms of IBS can be the source of considerable distress to a person with fibromyalgia due to the presence of abnormal sensory processing. In other words, because IBS causes abdominal discomfort and fibromyalgia causes pain amplification, a person with both conditions can experience severe visceral (intestinal) pain. Robert Bennett, M.D., suggests trying the following treatment options:

- Identify and eliminate foods that aggravate symptoms.

- Minimize stress.

- Adhere to basic rules for maintaining regular bowel habits, such as going at regular intervals and not delaying when you feel the urge to void (in cases of constipation)

- Use proper medications for specific symptoms:

  - Constipation: stool softener, fiber supplementation, and gentle laxatives such as bisacodyl

  - Diarrhea: loperamide or diphenoxylate

  - Antispasmodics: anticholinergics such as dicyclomine or hyoscyamine, or sedatives such as Donnatal or Librax

Mark Pimentel, M.D. and director of the Gastrointestinal Motility Program and Laboratory at Cedars-Sinai Medical Center, found that up to 80 percent of all IBS sufferers are affected by a condition called small intestinal bacterial overgrowth in which bacteria normally found in the lower gut colonizes the small intestine. The condition can be detected through a special breathalyzer test that typically checks for abnormal hydrogen levels after taking a dose of lactulose, which are indicative of the presence of bacterial overgrowth. The protocol is to reduce the bacteria through an extended treatment with a nonabsorbable antibiotic such as neomycin or rifaximin.

Pain Signal

A patient with both fibromyalgia and IBS has the ultimate catch-22. When the brain perceives pain, it tends to focus on the sensation and amplify it. An important practice to decrease the pain in both the gut and the entire body is to help the brain relax and focus on something else … such as floating on a cloud or swaying in a cool, soft breeze. Visualization can help calm the brain's desire to focus on the pain.

Cognitive Impairments: Fibro Fog

Cognitive problems such as impaired memory, poor concentration, and feelings of disorientation are common in people with fibromyalgia. These can be particularly difficult symptoms to deal with, especially when they interfere with your ability to remain employed.

Jennifer Glass, Ph.D., says, "Cognitive function can be thought of as the ability to carry out intellectual activities or processes, such as thinking, reasoning, remembering, imagining, or learning words. When the 'thinking' or 'remembering' actions seem faulty, completing simple daily tasks or job-related activities can become challenging and frustrating, no matter how familiar the activity."

def•i•ni•tion

Cognition is a broad term that refers to many different intellectual abilities and the different brain systems that support these abilities. Cognition involves the conscious process of knowing or being aware of thoughts and perceptions, including the ability to understand and reason.

In research studies at the University of Michigan, Glass and Denise Park, Ph.D., found that the cognitive performance of fibromyalgia patients was equivalent to that of adults who were 20 years older than them. However, on tests that evaluated *speed* of *cognition*, the people with fibromyalgia performed the same as those in their same age range. This seems to show that the cognitive problems associated with fibromyalgia are not the same as those that develop with age.

There are several types of systems that are involved in the process of memory. They include the following:

- **Working memory.** Combines short-term memory with other mental processes to enable us to "work things out in our heads." We use working memory when we do mental arithmetic.

- **Episodic memory.** Refers to the memory for particular episodes. An example is remembering what we were doing when we heard about the September 11 terrorist attacks.

- **Semantic memory.** Refers to our stored knowledge of facts, separate from any particular episodes associated with those facts. This is sometimes referred to as *declarative* memory.

The working and episodic memory systems of people with fibromyalgia, which combine short-term memory with other mental processes, were found to be less efficient than those without fibromyalgia who were the same age and had the same amount of education.

Park also found that the cognition problems are not associated with depression, because the fibromyalgia study participants were still able to perform at a relatively fast rate while those with depression were not. Although the exact reason why people with fibromyalgia have fibro fog is not known, it may have to do with the neuroendocrine abnormalities, sleep problems, mental fatigue, and chronic pain that, in turn, can affect the way our brains function. By treating these problems, you might also find relief from cognitive symptoms.

Migraine Headaches

Just as in the case of fibromyalgia, migraine headaches were once blamed on the ones who suffered from them. Today, there is more acceptance of this painful affliction, and new research is helping to find effective treatments.

Migraine headaches usually affect one side of the head and can last from a few hours to a few days. At the onset of a migraine, you might become sensitive to different types of stimulation, including lights, noises, or smells. You might begin to feel nauseated and start to vomit, and your head might feel like it is shrinking or caving in. Some people experience flashing lights or colors (called "migraine aura"), exhaustion, or even depression. These symptoms can continue throughout the migraine or give way to just the intense, piercing pain.

When a migraine begins, there are alterations in the blood flow to your brain, which contribute to the severe pain. It is thought that there may even be unusual electrical activity in the brain during a migraine headache.

Perhaps the best way to treat migraine headaches is to make every attempt to avoid having one. For instance, you should try to become aware of any food or environmental triggers that precipitate your migraines and then avoid them. If you are taking a prescription medication to treat your migraines, you should take the medication at the first sign of a migraine in order to limit the headache's severity. You can apply icepacks to your forehead, the back of your neck, or behind your knees. Lie down in a quiet, dark room and just rest. Do not try to watch TV or read.

A drop in your blood sugar can also trigger a migraine, so a small glass of fruit juice may help you feel better. Over-the-counter pain relievers may be helpful, and today there are dozens of prescription migraine medications that can be effective. In order to prevent migraines, some people benefit from taking beta-blockers (Inderal LA) or antiseizure medication (Depakote ER). For the treatment of migraine, other kinds of medications may be effective, including the triptans (such as Amerge, Imitrex, Zomig, Maxalt, and Axert), or a medication like Fioricet, which is a barbiturate sedative combined with a nonaspirin pain reliever (acetaminophen) and caffeine.

Healthy Alternative

To help reduce the number of migraines you might experience, try the following:

◆ Avoid using salt.

◆ Take aspirin along with an antinausea medication such as Reglan.

◆ Take a beta-blocker that relaxes blood vessels. These include Inderal, Corgard, Tenormin, Blocadren, and Toprol.

◆ Practice relaxation exercises.

◆ Use biofeedback to learn how to recognize pre-migraine symptoms, and then practice concentration techniques that will help lower your heart rate, blood pressure, and muscle tension.

Restless Legs Syndrome

Restless legs syndrome (RLS) is a disorder characterized by unusual sensations and strong urges to move your legs (and sometimes arms). These sensations usually occur in the evening either when you are trying to relax or when you lie down to sleep. These sensations in the legs can be described as creepy-crawly, itchy, pulling, nagging, and even painful. As you begin to rest, the symptoms become more pronounced and are accompanied by the desire to get up and walk, stretch, or move into another position. RLS can often be found in related family members. It can result in inadequate restorative sleep and cause you to feel tired and unrefreshed the next day.

People with RLS may also have *periodic limb movement disorder* (PLMD). This condition causes involuntary movement of the feet, legs, and arms while you are asleep. It can involve anything from small limited movements to wild and intense kicking and flailing of the legs and arms. The movements can be short in intensity or last up to 10 seconds.

 Pain Signal

Some people with RLS and PLMD experience a great deal of discomfort with muscles twitching or even violent leg and arm movements (where your extremities are flailing around without your control). Others, however, might not have such obvious symptoms. If your bed partner comments that you have a lot of leg or arm movement as you fall asleep, consider bringing this to your health-care provider's attention. You might be experiencing the negative effects of RLS/PLMD without even knowing it!

Proper treatment of RLS is typically determined on an individual basis. The first steps include identifying activities that worsen or improve the condition. If you walk, stretch, take a hot or cold bath or shower, perform acupressure, or rub your legs, you might be able to help relieve symptoms. Another option is to keep your mind busy by reading, doing arts or crafts, or even playing video games.

In some cases, RLS is associated with an underlying iron or vitamin deficiency (e.g., B_{12}) that can be treated by taking supplements. If these alternatives do not produce relief, there are four categories of medications that can be prescribed:

- **Dopaminergic agents.** Dopamine-receptor agonists approved for the treatment of RLS include Mirapex (pramipexole) and Requip (ropinirole). Drugs that add dopamine to the system may also be effective, such as Sinemet (carbidopa/levodopa). Although dopaminergic agents are used to treat Parkinson's disease, RLS is not a form of Parkinson's disease.

- **Sedative agents.** Sedatives are used either alone at bedtime or in addition to a dopaminergic agent. The most commonly used sedative is clonazepam (Klonopin).

- **Anticonvulsants.** People who have RLS daytime symptoms may be treated with the anticonvulsant gabapentin (Neurontin). This drug may be used if a pain condition is associated with the RLS.

- **Pain medications.** These agents are usually used only in extreme cases of RLS. Some examples of medications in this category include codeine, Darvon or Darvocet (propoxyphene), Dolophine (methadone), Percocet (oxycodone), Ultram (tramadol), and Vicodin (hydrocodone).

In addition, certain types of antidepressants (i.e., selective serotonin reuptake inhibitors, or SSRIs) are known either to cause or aggravate symptoms of RLS. Examples of SSRIs include Prozac (fluoxetine), Paxil (paroxetine), and Zoloft (sertraline). If you have RLS and are taking an SSRI, consider discussing a change in medication if you need treatment with an antidepressant. Examples of antidepressants that do not cause RLS include Wellbutrin SR/XL (bupropion extended-release) and EMSAM patch (transdermal selegiline).

Light/Sound Sensitivities

Just like pain amplification, sensory amplification (including adverse reactions to light and sound) is common in fibromyalgia. As a result of sensory overload, you might find that even minimal light and noise can cause distress. Weather changes can aggravate symptoms, and even light touch can be painful.

To be sensitive to something is to be responsive to a stimulus. People with fibromyalgia become ultrasensitive to a variety of stimuli that do not normally cause a negative reaction. To dilute the response to stimuli, you should avoid the situation, practice relaxation techniques, and avoid multitasking. Decreasing the amount of stimuli you are exposed to will help decrease the intensity of your reaction. Take things one at a time and make an effort to reduce the amount of environmental stressors you are exposed to.

Other Overlapping Conditions

Fibromyalgia is not limited to only the overlapping conditions that are discussed in this chapter. The majority of health-care providers treating fibromyalgia recognize up to 40 different related conditions. If you are affected by these other disorders, remember that there are treatment options, and if you and your health-care team focus on one or two problems at a time, you will have success in symptom reduction and even symptom elimination.

Fast Fact _____

In addition to the conditions discussed in this section, other common symptoms include …

♦ Diffuse numbness or tingling

♦ Jaw pain or discomfort ("TMJ")

♦ Painful menstrual periods

♦ Pain during intercourse

♦ Sensitivity to certain foods

♦ Frequent or painful urination

♦ Rapid heart rate and shortness of breath

♦ Sensation of swelling in hands and feet

♦ Ringing in the ears

♦ Rashes and dry skin

Keeping Track

In Appendix C, we include forms to track medications, complementary or alternative therapies, and treatments for overlapping conditions that you have already tried. There is also a space to indicate whether you found any of them to be helpful. Sharing this diary with your health-care provider may be beneficial when evaluating what course of treatment you wish to pursue.

Remember, resolving one symptom can also help improve or resolve another. Do not be overwhelmed. Again: knowledge is power, and armed with the knowledge you are gaining, you will better understand your illness and how to focus on the treatments that help you.

The Least You Need to Know

- If you can get relief from the symptoms of the overlapping conditions (such as headaches, migraines, IBS, dry mouth and eyes, restless legs, and so on), your fibromyalgia pain and fatigue can also becomes less pronounced.

- IBS, one of the most common overlapping conditions, causes abdominal discomfort, and because fibromyalgia causes pain amplification, a person with both syndromes can experience severe visceral (intestinal) pain.

- Cognitive performance of fibromyalgia patients has been shown to be equivalent to that of adults who were 20 years older than them.

- To reduce migraine headaches, you should become aware of food or environmental triggers and strive to avoid them.

- People with fibromyalgia become ultrasensitive to a variety of stimuli that normally do not cause a negative reaction in people who do not have the disorder.

Part 4

What Can I Do to Feel Better?

When it comes to improving your general well-being, you must look at yourself as a whole person. This means that you need to evaluate and implement activities that will improve the health of your body, mind, and soul. Your physical health will be impacted by your emotional health, and vice versa. If you view yourself as a "patient" rather than a person with fibromyalgia, you will be unable to move past your current situation to make the lifestyle changes that will help you to feel better and improve your overall quality of life.

In this part, you will learn that you can greatly improve how you feel just by keeping a positive attitude. When your emotional health improves, it will have a direct effect on your physical health. You can also feel better by improving your quantity and quality of sleep, becoming more physically active, and eating a healthy diet. Changes in how you feel can come about just by making small changes in your lifestyle and attitude.

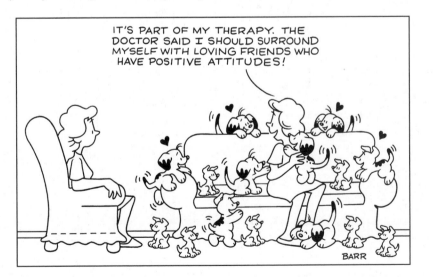

Emotional Health and Well-Being

In This Chapter

♦ Challenging emotions can affect your health

♦ Evaluating your psychological situation

♦ Having a positive attitude is important

♦ Understanding the mind-body connection

♦ Being prepared for a flare

Everyone faces emotional challenges in their lives. Death, divorce, loss of a job, and many other devastating occurrences can affect anyone. Although our initial emotional reactions to these events can be negative and intense, as time passes we learn to accept what has happened to us, and we learn how to move on. In the case of a chronic illness, however, the event that caused this initial negative emotional response does not go away. If we do not come to accept this new situation and learn how to focus on things besides the diagnosis of fibromyalgia, those intense emotions will stay with us. If your emotional self does not learn how to heal and accept, these negative emotions will continue to play a contributing role to your physical symptoms.

To feel better, you must recognize that there is a connection between your physical and emotional responses. Though you may have always been a positive person and coped well with adversity, you may need outside support to deal with the challenges that your diagnosis of fibromyalgia has brought you. Everyone can use emotional and physical support when they are dealing with a chronic illness. This chapter helps you learn how to better deal with your emotions—and what to expect after a diagnosis of fibromyalgia.

Diagnosis and Your Emotions

Before you were diagnosed with fibromyalgia, you probably worried about the cause of your symptoms, and wondered what was wrong with you. You might have even thought that you had cancer or a fatal illness. Experiencing pain is unnerving, but not knowing what is causing that pain can be extremely worrisome. After you received your diagnosis of fibromyalgia, you probably felt a great sense of relief. Finally you knew what was wrong. Although you have a complicated illness, it's not fatal. This can give you great peace of mind.

After this initial reaction, you may have questions such as, "What will my life with fibromyalgia be like?" The reality that you have a chronic illness can trigger a whole new set of fears. The first time you are invited to play tennis but you have to say no, or you are asked to chaperone your children's school outing but your pain prevents you from doing so, you realize how much your life has changed. Remember, however, that change doesn't have to be bad! It can make you feel confused and stressed until you become accustomed to your new situation. While you may feel blue or depressed at first, be aware that this emotional state can, in turn, cause a negative physical response. With fibromyalgia, stress accumulates and can build up to a point of extreme physical and emotional anxiety. It's impossible to live a stress-free life, so it is essential that you learn how to "de-stress" between stressful experiences. This includes learning how to implement the management tools that will help you identify and avoid stress accumulation and the threat of stress overload.

According to the American Academy of Family Physicians, it has been scientifically proven that your emotional state can affect your body and its physiological responses. When you get the flu and you wake up with a fever, headache, fatigue, and all-over pain, you just want to go to bed, pull the covers over your head, and sleep until the symptoms go away. You want to feel better as soon as possible! To accomplish this, you might take an over-the-counter pain reliever, a throat lozenge, and some extra vitamins—hoping that one of those treatments will make the illness go away. It's not surprising if you react to fibromyalgia the same way. You want your health-care professional to give you the magic pill that will allow you to go to bed for a few days and wake up feeling the way you did before you got sick. When the health-care professional tells you there is no magic pill, you may feel as though your life and health are out of your control. If you are not careful, negative emotions take over and cause you to spiral downward. When you are feeling bad emotionally, you will also feel worse physically.

Fast Fact

Stress can have both a positive and negative effect. Some types of stress can motivate and inspire us to accomplish great things. However, if excessive stress leaves you feeling overwhelmed, "tied up in knots," and exhausted, then you have not found the optimal stress level for your life. Remember that events or activities that were not stressful to you before fibromyalgia may now become the source of great amounts of stress. For example, something as simple as getting up in the middle of the night to go to the bathroom can now become a stressful situation. When you wake up, you may have several concerns: how difficult it is to move when you have been lying down and your body has become stiff, how unsteady you are on your feet, whether you'll be able to fall back to sleep, or whether you should turn on the light so you won't fall. An activity you had always taken for granted is now riddled with stress-provoking concerns.

Because there is such a connection between your feelings and your physical state, it is important to also address your psychological situation when you are creating your self-management plan. This does not mean that fibromyalgia is psychologically caused, but rather that any chronic illness will affect your emotions. To treat the whole person, it is imperative for patients to treat how they feel *both* psychologically and physically. The way you handle the entire experience is critical for achieving wellness. As you learned in previous chapters, when you get control of your situation and approach life in a more positive manner, your overall health will improve.

Pain Signal

Tara, one of the young public relations assistants working at the National Fibromyalgia Association, has fibromyalgia. One day she came into my office and burst into tears. For weeks her young cousin, who was living with an abusive parent, had been coming to her for help and advice. Tara explained that she was so worried about her young cousin that she felt exhausted, and her pain was becoming worse. She wanted to help, but she felt that the weight of her cousin's problems was adding to her fibromyalgia symptoms.

Stress Management Tools

The first step to living a more stress-free life is to identify your individual stressors and recognize their negative effects on your health. After you find the sources of your stress, you can work toward changing your reactions to these situations and/or managing them through change.

Picture This/Lessons Learned

Picture This:

When I was working at an advertising agency, I enjoyed going to a yoga class that was located just a few miles from my office building. I looked forward to my early evening classes and the joy and relaxation they brought to me. After years of attending classes in the same location, the yoga studio moved to a new building, in a different city, to accommodate more students. Class schedules were changed and my routine was rearranged. All of a sudden I found that I was driving a long distance to attend a class scheduled later in the day. My favorite teacher no longer taught there, and my formerly relaxing yoga classes were now emotionally and physically stressful.

Lessons Learned:

It took me a while to realize that my "relaxing yoga classes" were now stressful occurrences. Even though I enjoyed yoga, I was becoming stressed by the events surrounding the actual activity. The longer drive, the later class schedule, and even the new teacher made the experience stressful. To avoid the stress, I realized that I needed to find a class in a more convenient location, at a time that fit my schedule. I also needed to open my mind to a new teacher. By eliminating the stressors and by becoming accepting of a new teacher, I once again found my yoga classes to be joyful and relaxing!

There are many options for managing stress. If you find yourself identifying certain circumstances or activities as stressful, ask yourself the following questions:

♦ What is causing you to feel stress? Is it something that should not normally be stressful?

♦ When you are feeling stressed, how does your body react? Are you having physical reactions such as tight muscles, stomachaches, and headaches?

♦ Is it possible to eliminate whatever is causing your stress? Can you learn to say no, change a habit, or avoid the stressor?

- Is it possible to reduce your exposure to whatever is causing your stress? If you only have to do something once a week, rather than every day, it might not be as stressful.

- Is it possible to vary or change the situation that is causing your stress? Modifying a stressor can mean anything from turning the radio down to changing jobs or even moving.

- Can you rest or relax after exposure to a certain stressor? If you have to work in a stressful situation, can you take breaks to lie down and rest, allowing your body to restore itself?

- Can you change the environment that is causing stress? Are there certain people or situations you need to avoid?

- Can you change your attitude toward whatever is causing you stress? Would eliminating negative thoughts be helpful?

- Have you put too much pressure on yourself? Are your expectations for yourself realistic?

- Do you get stuck on "yes, buts," and "what ifs"? Can you concentrate on the present and the immediate future, instead of worrying about the distant future?

- Can you practice relaxation exercises such as slow rhythmic breathing, meditation practices, or visualization?

- If you are experiencing stress, can you do something to relieve the stress? Try to get more sleep, exercise, eat better, or do more things that you enjoy.

- If you are stressed about a situation, do you have people that you can call on to help you?

For more information on stress-related issues, please refer to Chapter 17.

What Is the Mind-Body Connection?

There are very different ideas about approaching the mind-body connection. You have no doubt experienced aspects of the mind-body connection and have seen this phenomenon at work—making you less healthy or more healthy. For example, if you're in school and stay up all night studying for a big test, the stress you experience enables you to go without sleep. After the test is over and you begin to relax, the energy you felt while studying turns to exhaustion, and you may even get sick. Or if you are not feeling well and your best friend comes over and makes you laugh, you may feel better. In the practice of holistic medicine, the focus is on the importance of inner peace and calm, freeing the body to function more efficiently.

Those who look for a more scientific explanation for the mind-body connection point to psychological reactions that happen without our control. We know that when we have an emotional feeling, it can cause the body to react in a specific way. If you become frightened, your body might begin to shake; or if you are embarrassed, your face might turn red. These reactions happen because your emotions cause certain neurons within the hypothalamus of the brain to convert the *neural impulses* of your thoughts and emotions into hormonal information that makes the body react. Can you control your thoughts, therefore controlling the effect they have on your physical reactions? Currently there is much research delving into this subject. Richard J. Davidson, Ph.D., of the University of Wisconsin, continues to study the mechanisms of mind-body interaction with an emphasis on emotion as a core influence on your health. Today, more attention has turned to understanding the power of the mind.

def•i•ni•tion

> **Neural impulses,** or neural transmissions, are a basic function to the nervous system, sending signals between neurons. The sympathetic nervous system (part of the autonomic nervous system) dominates in stressful situations and prepares the body for a physical response—it's called the "fight or flight" response. For example, if you feel as though you are in physical danger, your heart will beat faster and you will get a rush of adrenaline or energy. In a stressful situation that doesn't require a physical response, the sympathetic nervous system will cause your body to react in the same way.

Maintaining balance is one way a person with fibromyalgia can feel better. Maintaining a balanced life can help you manage your energy and stress levels; maintaining a balanced outlook is vital when you consider potential treatments, and even when you take a look at your mind's impact on your health. If you start to think, "I can heal myself by willing it to happen," you may experience more frustration if your efforts don't produce the results you want. On the other hand, there *is* a connection between the mind and the body. Without focusing on emotional health and a healthy attitude, you will decrease your odds of physical improvement. The bottom line is what you think will have an effect on your total health. Each influences the other.

Fast Fact _____

Dr. Richard Davidson has found that with today's brain imaging techniques, it is possible to learn how individual differences in the activation levels in different parts of the brain can play an important role in regulating specific responses to emotional events. In other words, the brain's biochemistry actually affects what the emotional response will be in a given situation. For more information, go to www.loc.gov/loc/brain/emotion/Davidson.html.

Power of Positive Thinking

Some people tend to be naturally more persistent, better at problem solving, and more open to change. This group of people often has an easier time thinking positive thoughts. The good news, however, is that everyone can learn how to think more positively. If you can recognize your negative thoughts and learn how to identify what makes you think that way, you can focus on turning those thoughts into positive ones. Your positive thoughts can help you find solutions to make coping easier. It is important to know that even with chronic illness, healing and symptom improvement is always possible.

Dr. Dennis Turk, director of the Fibromyalgia Research Center and professor of anesthesiology and pain research at the University of Washington, has identified categories of negative thinking. If you can evaluate your way of thinking and can identify negative thoughts, you can establish a pattern of positive thinking that will relieve stress and emotional suffering, and help you move forward. Dr. Turk warns that changing the negative thinking habit takes time and practice.

The following chart can help you identify negative thought patterns.

Category	Definition	Example
Blaming	You make someone or something else responsible for your pain.	"It's my boss's fault that I am stressed and in pain."
	You think it is your fault.	"I am so dumb. It is no wonder I got sick."
"Should" statements	Implies you did not do the right thing.	"I should have been nicer to my husband."
Polarized thinking	Things are either black or white.	"I have FM so I will never have a happy life."
Catastrophizing	Involves saying "what if."	"What if my husband leaves me?"
Control fallacies	Thinking that others have complete dependence on you and control over you.	"Everyone depends on me and the family will fall apart if I am sick."
Emotional	If you feel something, it must be true. You let your emotions rule your ability to reason.	"I feel like I am going to die, so it must be true."
Filtering	You only hear negative things, not positive ones.	"The health-care professional said there is no treatment." (What was actually said: "There is no treatment that cures FM, but there are lots of things we can try.")
Entitlement fallacy	You want life to give you only the best. You believe life should be fair.	"Because I am a good person, this should not be happening to me!"

Reframing for Positive Thoughts

Reframing is changing the way you react to and interpret a situation (for example, if you see the glass as half-full, rather than half-empty). If you start to think a negative thought, such as, "Everything bad happens to me," or "I don't deserve anything better," recognize that thought, and make yourself turn it into a positive one. If you think, "Today is going to be a bad day," stop and make yourself think, "Today will be a good day." Eventually your attitude will change to match your way of thinking. Even if you don't always believe the more positive thought, by forcing yourself to recognize your negative thinking and turning it into a more positive thought, over time you will see the improvement in your life and health.

Use reframing to monitor your thoughts and to establish the positive thinking habit. This process will help you be more positive in situations where you were previously reacting negatively. By repeating this exercise multiple times, you will gradually change your negative thinking habits. Eventually you will automatically react to things in a more positive way.

Positive Thought Worksheet

Following is an exercise to help you practice making your thoughts more positive. It is called the "Positive Thought Worksheet."

When you have a negative reaction to an experience, write it down and rank how negative your reaction was. Evaluate the negative reaction in writing, and think about how you can make your thoughts more positive. After you have come up with a more positive reaction, evaluate how positive your final thought was. If you practice doing this throughout the day, you will begin to automatically think more positively!

Here is an example:

Event: *My husband was mad at me for not doing the dishes when I was in pain.*

Your thoughts/reactions to the event: *I hate myself because I have this illness and I am not a good wife. It makes me feel less useful and causes problems between my husband and me.*

Rank your thoughts 1–10 (1 = negative; 10 = positive): *3*

List aspects of your thoughts that were negative: *I blame myself for my illness and I feel like I am less valuable. I blame my illness for my disagreements with my husband.*

Evaluate the negative thoughts: *This illness is not my fault. I didn't do the dishes because I felt it was healthier for me to rest, and so I won't be in as much pain tomorrow. I am not less of a person because I have FM, I just need to adjust my priorities. My husband and I had a few disagreements like this before I was sick.*

List how your thoughts could become more positive: *My reaction could have been less hard on myself. The comment could have led the way for me to explain my actions to my husband and help him understand and accept my illness.*

What is your final positive thought? *I am pleased with myself for recognizing that I was in too much pain to do the dishes and that by resting I won't be in as much pain tomorrow. I will explain this to my husband. I will thank him for helping me today and assure him that I will help him with one of his tasks as soon as I feel better.*

Rank your final thoughts 1–10 (1 = negative; 10 = positive): _9_

Now you can practice becoming more positive. Make copies of the following Positive Thought Worksheet and use it as needed until thinking more positively becomes natural to you.

Event:

_____

_____

Your thoughts/reactions to the event:

_____

_____

_____

Rank your thoughts 1–10 (1 = negative; 10 = positive): ____

List aspects of your thoughts that were negative:

_____

_____

Evaluate the negative thoughts:

_____

_____

_____

List how your thoughts could become more positive:

_____

_____

_____

What is your final positive thought?

_____

_____

_____

Rank your final thoughts 1–10 (1 = negative; 10 = positive): ____

Managing the Ups and Downs of Fibromyalgia

The ups and downs, or waxing and waning, of fibromyalgia symptoms are both physically and emotionally draining. It is not unusual for intense pain to drain your energy, making it difficult to do the things necessary to stay emotionally positive. When your symptoms become more intense, not only will you need to concentrate on the medical treatments that will get you through the flare, but you must also focus on the behaviors that keep your mind positive. The minute your symptoms become more aggravated, it is imperative that you implement a slate of predetermined activities to assist you with coping. If you have a plan in place, it will take much less energy and time to move away from destructive thoughts to a mind-set that will be emotionally beneficial. It is often tempting to figure out what brought on the flare, but because flare-ups may occur with no identifiable cause, this can be a fruitless and negative exercise.

Healthy Alternative

When you experience a flare-up of your fibromyalgia symptoms, it is important to concentrate on what you can do rather than what you can't do. Keep a list of things that make your feel better so you can quickly undertake an activity that has helped in the past. This list might include things such as: talk to my doctor about increasing my medications; place a cold cloth on my head and close my eyes to rest; schedule a massage; have my husband read to me; sleep in the other room, where it is cooler and less noisy; listen to my favorite CD and relax; drink more water to make sure I am not dehydrated; avoid all products that contain caffeine; or talk to my friend who is always a positive influence on me.

Actions for Emotional Coping With Flares

Here are some other ideas you can implement the next time your symptoms become severe. Be sure to add your own ideas to this list, and refer to it to help you get through the emotionally rough times.

◆ Imagine yourself in a peaceful, happy place. Visualize the specifics of this harmonious place. Visit this place in your mind whenever you feel down emotionally.

◆ Attend a fibromyalgia support-group meeting. Do not complain about how you feel, but rather socialize with others who understand what you are going through.

◆ Visit a counselor or spiritual minister. Listen, as well as share. Let people be there for you.

◆ Repeat the following: "I will feel better than I feel right now."

◆ Change your environment. Go to a place that makes you feel happy. It could be another room in your house, a chair in your yard, a friend's house, the park, or out of town. Give yourself a new perspective.

◆ Put together a box of items that have happy memories. These may include a letter from a dear friend, a doll from your childhood, a book of poems, a painting your child made you, your favorite photos, or a shell you collected while on vacation. Enjoy these memories, and know that you will have more special memories in the future.

◆ Create a comfort zone. (Have a member of your family help if necessary.) Change the sheets on your bed, use as many pillows as you need, wear your most comfortable clothing, use a heating pad or ice pack, have your favorite drink by your side, put on relaxing music, suck on ice chips, place a cool cloth on your forehead, or place aromatic herbs or potpourri in your pillowcase.

◆ Watch or read something that makes you laugh. Practice smiling.

◆ Call on your support team. Having others tell you that things are going to get better can help you believe it is true.

◆ Take time to relax, breathe deeply, and heal.

Who Am I Now—a Patient or a Person?

Although you have an illness and are considered a patient when you see a medical practitioner, it is important to avoid taking on the persona of "patient," rather than "person." If you view yourself as only a patient, you are defining yourself based on your illness. Fibromyalgia is an illness you have, not the person you are. If you think of yourself as a patient, you will ignore your symptom improvements. You will be *stuck* in this place of affliction, never allowing yourself to accept and adjust to the changes in your life. Remember that you are who you are, not what you do—and certainly not what illness you have.

 Pain Signal _____

Who you are is *not* defined by your fibromyalgia. If you were a good person before you got sick, you are still a good person. If you were a smart person before you got sick, you are still a smart person. If you were a compassionate person before you got sick, you are still a compassionate person. If you were a mean person before you got sick, let's hope that you have become a compassionate person!

The Least You Need to Know

- The reality that you have a chronic illness can trigger a whole new set of fears.

- After you find the sources of your stress, you can work toward changing your reactions to these situations and/or managing them through change.

- Having an emotional feeling can cause your body to react in a specific way.

- Reframing is changing the way you react to and interpret a situation.

- When you are experiencing a flare-up of your fibromyalgia symptoms, it is important to concentrate on what you can do, rather than what you can't do.

- Fibromyalgia is an illness you have, not the person you are.

Chapter 15

Healthy Lifestyle Changes: Sleep

In This Chapter

- ◆ Changing your lifestyle is important
- ◆ Recognizing and accepting that change is good
- ◆ Understanding which lifestyle changes are necessary
- ◆ Understanding sleep hygiene
- ◆ Learning how to change your sleep habits
- ◆ Learning how to relax

One of the most important things you can do to improve your overall health is to recognize which aspects of your lifestyle need to change so you can avoid aggravating your fibromyalgia symptoms. Fibromyalgia results in increased sensitivity to pain, sound, light, and other stimuli. To help decrease this hypersensitivity, you need to become hardier, healthier, and stronger. Some of the modifications you need to make involve your attitude, whereas others focus on your behaviors. In this chapter, you learn that making changes to your lifestyle can have wonderful rewards, both physically and emotionally. For instance, it is possible to change your sleep habits so that you can enjoy a much more restful night's sleep. After you accept that change is a good thing, you will be on your way to finding new ways to live a happier and healthier life!

Evaluating Your Lifestyle

The word "change" often excites anxiety, hostility, and fear. We are creatures of habit, and when someone suggests a different way of doing things, we may feel unsettled about moving out of our comfort zone. But "change" doesn't have to mean "bad" or "unfair"! In fact, change can help us develop appropriate coping behaviors, help reduce stress, and restore a sense of order and purpose to our lives.

Picture This/Lessons Learned

Picture This:

When I was a teenager, my father was diagnosed with multiple sclerosis (MS) and my family's way of life had to completely change. My mother became the primary financial supporter, my brother and I had to accept more responsibility in caring for the house, and we all had to help care for my father. Nothing was the same and it all seemed terribly unfair—but it was worth it to help my father.

Lessons Learned:

Although my father's MS placed him immediately in a wheelchair and he spent 16 years almost completely bedfast, he never gave up hope. Near the end of his life, he told my mother that the reason he fought so hard to stay alive was his family's willingness to adapt to his new situation. It assured him that we loved him a lot. If we were willing to do this for him, he wanted to do everything he could to show us his appreciation. I believe that my father had an additional motivation to live a happy life, despite his illness, because of my family's willingness to work together and make changes to our lifestyle.

You can choose to resist necessary change, or you can learn to accept it. Often, valuable energy is wasted by worrying about change rather than taking positive action to embrace it enthusiastically and creatively. Developing a healthier lifestyle is a process you can enjoy and be proud of—and if you approach this change one step at a time, the process need not be painful or arduous.

It's important to set realistic goals and make gradual changes. If you are willing to work through some initial emotional discomfort as you ease into a new lifestyle, you'll find the confidence, dedication, and determination to ensure a smooth transition. After you start achieving great results, the improvements you experience will make you willing—maybe even eager—to institute additional positive changes. And enjoying the wonderful benefits of a healthy lifestyle will encourage you to stick with the changes that have already positively impacted how you feel.

So what kinds of changes are you going to make? Most people with fibromyalgia led productive, active lives before they developed fibromyalgia. They are often hard-working people who led fast-paced lives, neglecting their own health. They usually are not comfortable asking others for help, and they like to stay busy. Many of these characteristics are not compatible with the symptoms of fibromyalgia.

Certain changes are necessary for you to adapt to a healthier lifestyle that will not inflame your symptoms. Some of the changes you implement will be temporary, and others will be permanent. As you start to feel better, you may realize that you do not need to stick with some of the changes you have made—but you may just discover that this new way of approaching life brings you more pleasure than your old way of doing things.

Healthy Alternative

Change does not necessarily mean that you have to give something up. Sometimes all you have to do is make an adjustment. For example, if gardening is your passion but it has become too painful for you to do, you can still enjoy gardening by modifying the way you approach it. Plant hanging baskets and flower boxes so that you don't have to bend over so much. Fill your yard with low-maintenance plants and spend more time smelling the flowers than weeding them!

Lifestyle Changes

The following are examples of some changes that you should consider to establish a lifestyle compatible with fibromyalgia. Later in this chapter, you will have an opportunity to develop and prioritize your individual lifestyle changes.

- Improve your sleep habits.

- Exercise at least a small amount every day.

- Change your diet to include healthier foods.

- Learn how to relax and enjoy quiet, self-reflection time.

- Conserve personal energy. Set realistic goals.

- Eliminate foods and activities that are not healthy, such as caffeine and tobacco use.

◆ Shift your focus and establish new priorities.

◆ Make sense out of your life's new purpose.

◆ Take part in activities that focus on your emotional well-being.

Some of the changes you make will be up to your discretion. However, there are some changes that have been shown to be important in improving fibromyalgia symptoms. Learning how to change your sleep habits, exercise routine, diet, and the pace of your life, as well as finding ways to save energy, will be crucial to symptom reduction. Establishing and sticking to a routine that works for you will be invaluable. But remember, the process must be gradual.

Personal Lifestyle Change Goals

As you read about lifestyle changes, make a list of the ones you believe you need to make. These will become your personal lifestyle change goals.

Even though each change may seem simple, it can be difficult to let go of doing things the way you always have. Take it slowly and remember that with each change, you are improving your health. Some of the changes that I decided to make were …

◆ Drink more water each day so I'm not dehydrated.

◆ Ask my husband for help when I need something heavy to be moved or lifted.

◆ Leave things at the foot of the stairs so I don't have to go up and down the stairs so many times in one day.

◆ Get help rearranging my office so it is more ergonomic.

◆ Stop wearing high-heeled shoes because they leave my legs and feet aching.

◆ My husband cooks dinner so I can rest and recuperate from a day of work.

Improve Your Sleep

Sleep is something most people take for granted—until they experience the frustrations and symptoms that accompany insufficient or only poor-quality sleep. Lying in bed awake at night or waking up feeling unrefreshed and exhausted can be as big a challenge as managing pain.

Many health-care professionals believe that if you improve your quantity and quality of sleep, you will reduce other fibromyalgia symptoms. For this reason, it is important to learn about proper sleep hygiene and be sure that your sleep disturbances are not being caused by other medical conditions, such as restless legs syndrome, sleep apnea, acid reflux, or narcolepsy.

Are You Sleeping or Counting Sheep?

While it may seem that you are either sleeping or awake, there are really four levels of sleep you should be going through each night as you rest. For those with fibromyalgia, though, reaching the deep stages of sleep can be difficult, preventing you from getting the restorative sleep you need.

The four stages of sleep are as follows:

- ◆ **Stage 1:** This is when a person moves from being awake to falling asleep. They become less aware of their surroundings, and as their breathing becomes more relaxed and regular, they begin to experience rolling eye movement. This stage of sleep only accounts for about 5 percent of total sleep time.

- ◆ **Stage 2**: This is the first stage of true sleep, even though it is a light sleep from which it is easy to be aroused. Stage 2 sleep accounts for about 50 percent of total sleep. An individual usually spends about 30 minutes in stage 2 sleep.

- ◆ **Stages 3 and 4:** This period is referred to as slow wave sleep. As a person moves into a very relaxed state, his heartbeat and respiratory rate become slow and regular. His muscles become more relaxed, and it is difficult to awaken him. On average, an adult spends about 7 percent of his total sleep time in stage 3, and around 11 percent in stage 4. The body is believed to carry out most of its repair work during these stages of sleep.

- ◆ **REM (rapid eye movement):** Discovered in 1953, REM sleep was identified as an active period of sleep in which a person's eyes move in a rapid, flickering, twitching motion while the eyelids are closed. It was also discovered that during REM sleep, a person is likely to dream. REM sleep is experienced within 90 minutes of falling asleep. It recurs about every 90 minutes throughout the night, and each time it recurs, the individual spends a little bit longer in this stage.

So what is a normal night of sleep? Most people spend the majority of the night in stage 1, which is transitioning between being awake and asleep, and stage 2, which is the first stage of light sleep. It isn't until stages 3 and 4 that the body is able to achieve a level of sleep that is restorative and refreshing. In stage 4, growth hormones and other chemicals are released for essential body tissue repair. After reaching stage 4, the deepest period of sleep, the pattern reverses and sleep becomes progressively lighter until REM sleep occurs.

Scientists have found that in REM (rapid eye movement) sleep, the body is paralyzed and the individual experiences an active, dreamlike state. People with normal sleep patterns usually spend about two hours a night in REM sleep, whereas people with fibromyalgia often spend hours in this "dreamy" level of sleep. Studies have found that when people with fibromyalgia reach the deeper levels of sleep (slow wave sleep), *alpha brain waves* intrude and jolt them back into shallow sleep. Therefore, although they spend hours in REM sleep, they are not able to sustain the deep stages of restorative sleep that are necessary to achieve the recuperative benefits sleep is supposed to provide.

def•i•ni•tion

Alpha brain waves were first discovered around 1908 by an Austrian psychiatrist named Hans Berger. Alpha waves are seen in a wakeful state of consciousness when the individual experiences a relaxed and effortless alertness. The brains of creative people can generate bursts of these alpha waves to help them with problem-solving. The opposite state of alpha waves are delta waves, which are present when a person is in the deepest stages of sleep.

Nonrestorative Sleep Leaves You Exhausted

Individuals with fibromyalgia have a variety of problems associated with sleep, but it all comes down to one thing: they experience nonrestorative sleep. Even after being in bed all night, most people with fibromyalgia wake up feeling unrefreshed. It is important to keep a natural sleep rhythm to facilitate the secretion of hormones such as cortisol, growth hormone, and melatonin. The cycles of these hormones become disrupted if you are not able to fall asleep until the early hours of the morning (delayed sleep phase disorder) or if you cannot stay asleep throughout the night (fitful sleep disorder). These sleep disturbances can be caused by napping during the day or lack of physical activity. People with fibromyalgia can also be awakened by restless legs syndrome, cramps, shortness of breath, and pain. Whatever the cause of the sleep disturbances, the lack of restorative sleep will be associated with fatigue and increased pain.

Pain Signal

Many sleep disorders go undiagnosed. If you experience unrefreshed sleep, talk to your health-care professional and find out if you might benefit from an evaluation by a reputable sleep center. In some cases you will be asked to spend the night at the center, but in other cases the testing equipment can be brought to your home.

One of the major consequences of nonrestorative sleep is fatigue. The fatigue associated with fibromyalgia and chronic fatigue syndrome goes beyond exhaustion. It can cause poor concentration, memory loss, anxiety, and the inability to perform even basic tasks. It is necessary to combat fatigue with a program that will help reestablish healthier sleep.

Good Sleep Hygiene—Getting Your ZZZs

Sleep hygiene is a term used to define proper sleep habits that result in normal, quality nighttime sleep and daytime alertness. The goal is to maintain a regular sleep-and-wake pattern, seven days a week. This means that you need to implement the same routine during the week and on weekends, so that you sleep between seven and a half and eight hours per night. Some fibromyalgia patients have difficulty sleeping even a few hours within a 24-hour period, whereas others are so exhausted that they sleep all day long and then are wide awake at night. Whichever issue you are dealing with, it's important to go to sleep and get up at the same time every day.

It is also important to get an appropriate number of continuous hours of sleep each night: not too many, and not too few. By setting a stable pattern for your sleep, you help reset your biological clock. In humans, the biological clock controls temperature and hormone synthesis patterns, and even an overall state of equilibrium. When it is disturbed, it can bring about illness and sleep disorders.

Fast Fact

Seven and a half to eight hours of sleep is the average amount of sleep that most adults require. Remember, everyone is different. The goal is to sleep continuously for the same amount of time each night, which will make you feel refreshed in the morning and throughout the next day.

The following are ways you can increase good sleep hygiene:

♦ Attempt to do regular exercise every day. Because exercise warms your body and a decreased body temperature is a sign to go to sleep, be sure you don't exercise close to the time you are going to bed.

♦ Avoid taking naps during the day. If you must take a nap, do not sleep for more than 30 minutes total. Rest periods, when you sit or lie down for 10 minutes without falling asleep, may help to restore your energy when you become tired during the day.

♦ Establish a routine of going to bed and waking up at approximately the same time every day. Establishing regularity in your sleep patterns will make your body perform better.

♦ When you go to bed, it should be for rest, sleep, or intimacy only. Avoid watching TV in bed or discussing stressful subjects before you go to sleep.

♦ If you have trouble falling asleep, do not drink caffeinated beverages, eat chocolate, or smoke cigarettes. These stimulants can prevent you from getting deep, quality sleep.

♦ Alcohol can also fragment your sleep. Although you may have heard that it will help you *get* to sleep, the problem begins when the body starts to metabolize the alcohol, waking you up and fragmenting your night's sleep.

♦ Talk to your health-care professional about your medications (over-the-counter and prescription) and whether what you are taking may be acting as a stimulant. Avoid unnecessary medications with alertness side effects. Discuss whether an herbal sleep aid, such as Calms Forte, is appropriate, or if a prescription for sleeping pills is right for you. The decision to take sleeping aids is a medical one that should be made in consideration of your overall health situation.

♦ Reduce environmental factors that may prevent you from falling asleep or that arouse you from sleep:

  ♦ Get into a position that is comfortable for you to fall asleep.

  ♦ Make sure your bed is comfortable. (Additional padding can soften the mattress to your liking.)

  ♦ Make sure your pillows are comfortable. Use extra pillows to prop up areas that are especially sore. Consider using a water-filled pillow that can help support your neck.

- ◆ Make sure the room is not too hot or cold. Avoid extreme temperatures.

- ◆ Protect the room from external noises and bright light. Disconnect the phone and use earplugs or eyeshades if necessary, and install blackout shades to help reduce outside light.

- ◆ Decorate your bedroom to make it a relaxing place. Don't paint the walls with bright colors or jam it full of furniture and clutter. Computers and exercise machines belong in other areas of the house.

- ◆ Although some people need complete silence to fall asleep, others find white noise soothing. Examples of white noise include a fan, a waterfall, or the humming of a machine.

- ◆ Hide your bedroom clock from your view. If you wake up in the middle of the night, don't look at the time. If you know what time it is, you may feel anxious about how much or how little time there is left for sleeping.

- ◆ Avoid eating a meal right before bedtime. Do not go to bed too full or too hungry, and be careful of what you eat in the evening. Certain foods can cause heartburn or gas that can disrupt sleep. It may be helpful to drink a glass of milk or eat a small portion of turkey or other foods that contain the amino acid tryptophan, which can help induce sleep.

◆ If possible, make sure that you are not the person responsible for taking care of children or pets when you are trying to go to sleep. To know that someone else is taking care of these responsibilities will help you feel more relaxed.

◆ Establish a bedtime routine:

- ◆ Avoid emotionally upsetting conversations and activities before trying to go to sleep.

- ◆ Take care of health-related activities, such as washing your face, brushing your teeth, and taking your medications.

- ◆ Do something relaxing to calm your mind and body, such as meditation or reading something light and entertaining. Listen to soft music with your eyes closed.

◆ If you cannot fall asleep after 20 minutes, get out of bed and do something besides trying to fall asleep. Concentrate on the pleasant sensation of relaxing. Don't expose yourself to bright light while you are out of bed because this will wake you up instead of helping you fall asleep.

◆ When you get up in the morning, make sure you expose yourself to a lot of sunlight before 9 A.M. Light exposure helps maintain your circadian rhythm. You do not have to sunbathe; just get out into the sunlight.

Things to Do at Bedtime

Creating bedtime rituals will help cue your body that it is time to slow down and relax, and can help you get to sleep faster. Here are some rituals to try:

◆ Sipping a cup of herbal tea, reading poetry, writing in a journal, getting a soft massage, doing breathing exercises, meditating, enjoying quiet time with your pet, sitting in a room lit only by candlelight, or saying a prayer.

◆ Having a small glass of warm milk before going to bed. Not only is it soothing, but the warmth may temporarily increase your body temperature and the subsequent drop may bring on sleep.

◆ Taking a warm shower or bath before bed. This is an excellent way to soothe sore muscles and bring on a sense of calm and relaxation.

◆ Making sure that you go to the bathroom right before you get into bed. This is important so you won't have to get up in the middle of the night.

◆ Making a list of things you want to deal with or accomplish the next day and then setting the list aside, knowing that you don't have to think about these things throughout the night. Leave your worries about job, school, daily life, and so on behind when you go to bed.

The Sleep-Hygiene Test

The following sleep-hygiene test will help you evaluate your current level of appropriate sleep behaviors. Rank how often you do the following activities on a scale of 1 to 5, with 1 being never and 5 being always.

Sleep Hygiene Test

Rank	Activity
_____	I take a long nap in the afternoon.
_____	I go to bed after midnight on the weekends.

Rank	Activity
_____	When I wake up in the middle of the night, I stay in bed and toss and turn.
_____	When I get home from my daily activities, I eat and then immediately go to bed.
_____	My computer is in my bedroom, and I often send and read e-mails right before I go to bed.
_____	My bedroom is always very cold at night because my spouse does not like a room that is warm.
_____	I wake up two to three times a night to get something to drink, check on the kids, or go to the bathroom.
_____	I get a second wind after dinner and find all sorts of challenging projects to do.
_____	I like to have a glass of wine or a drink before I go to bed because it helps me sleep.
_____	After I get into bed, I think about all the things I have to do the next day.

The behaviors in this sleep hygiene test reflect poor sleep habits. If your test score total was more than 20 points, you need to work on improving your sleep habits. Scores between 15 and 20 indicate that there is room for improvement in your sleep hygiene routine.

Fast Fact

In studies where medical students were deprived of sleep, they developed many symptoms similar to those of fibromyalgia. Sleep deprivation can cause symptoms beyond fatigue, including cognitive difficulties, pain, and anxiety.

Personal Sleep Plan

You can make changes on your own, but you may also want to consult a behavior-modification therapist or visit a sleep center. If your sleep habits are still not conducive to good sleep, develop a plan to make positive changes to your sleep hygiene.

Rule Out Other Medical Conditions

While sleep problems are a prominent symptom of fibromyalgia, it is important to rule out other medical conditions that can also aggravate sleep. If you answer "yes" to any of the following questions, bring these symptoms to the attention of your medical health-care professional. If they are part of a condition other than fibromyalgia, your health-care professional can treat the problem properly.

◆ Do you have muscle spasms or find that your legs or arms jump or twitch throughout the night? When sitting or lying down, do you have a strong, nearly irresistible urge to move your legs? You may have restless legs syndrome.

◆ Does your own snoring wake you up? Do you ever wake up with the feeling that you cannot breathe? You may have sleep apnea. A sleep study will help identify the problem, which can then be treated.

◆ Do you wake up with parts of your body feeling numb or asleep? You may have blood-vessel constriction.

◆ Do you wake up because you have pain and burning in your stomach or chest area? You may have Gastro Esophageal Reflux Disease, or GERD.

◆ Do you have trouble sleeping because you feel life is out of your control? You may be dealing with depression or anxiety.

◆ Are you obese? Obesity is associated with sleep disturbances.

◆ Do you fall asleep easily during the day and sometimes in inappropriate situations? You may have narcolepsy.

◆ Do you sleep all day and then find yourself awake all night? You are experiencing alpha waves at night and delta waves during the day—the opposite of a typical circadian rhythm.

If you answered yes to any of these questions, make sure you consult with your health-care professional.

Learn How to Relax

An active lifestyle can be rewarding and interesting, but unless you take time to relax, you will increase your symptoms of muscle tension and pain, sleep problems, an overactive mind which can lead to anxiety, and even the inability to concentrate and appreciate the world around you. If you always focus on keeping your mind active and ignore your body, eventually you will find yourself physically *and* emotionally unhealthy. It's important to maintain balance. Everyone should schedule some time each day to slow down, take it easy, relax, reflect, and enjoy. This means that you must intentionally rest both your body and your mind.

You can practice relaxing in many different ways. You may want to take some time to sit quietly, empty your mind of active thoughts, and imagine a peaceful, calm place. Lie down, focusing on the slow rhythm of your breathing, allowing all the stress and tension to slip from your mind and body. You can use a certain sound (such as the sound of a siren or a loud noise) or a specific place (whenever you stop at a red light while driving your car) to remind you to take time to relax, breathe, and reflect on the beautiful things around you. You may want to schedule a specific time each day to perform a relaxation exercise to help you relax your body and mind.

Relaxation Exercise #1

Lie down on a bed and make sure that you are well supported and comfortable. The room should be quiet and dark, and have a pleasant temperature. Take a couple of deep slow breaths, letting go of the tension that you feel in your body.

Start by visualizing your entire body lying comfortably on the bed. Then think about your toes. Wiggle them, and then tense and relax them; say to yourself, "Toes, relax and disappear." In your mind, picture your body without toes. Next, tense and relax your feet. Again, say to yourself, "Feet, relax and disappear." This time when you visualize your body, picture your body without your toes or the bottom portion of your feet. Repeat this process, moving up your body and making your legs, thighs, buttocks, hips, stomach, back, chest, hands, arms, neck, and head tighten up, relax, and then disappear. Finally, visualize your spirit floating throughout the universe, completely relaxed and totally carefree. Enjoy the feeling of lightness and freedom.

Relaxation Exercise #2

Lie down on a bed or sit comfortably in a chair. Close your eyes and let go of all concerns, turbulent thoughts, and fears. Let your body go limp, allowing your muscles and bones to relax into the bed or chair. Visualize your body light as a cloud, relaxing any part of your body that still feels tense. Take some time to relax and just *be*, recognizing how wonderful it is to feel light and relaxed.

Then visualize yourself exactly where you are. Imagine your body rising off that piece of furniture and starting to float upward. Repeat to yourself, "I am lighter than air." Continue to visualize your body floating higher and higher, until you are floating above the building you were in. Keep thinking of floating upward, repeating the words, "I am lighter than air." Picture yourself floating above your city, your state, your country, the world, and the universe, until you are floating out to infinity.

Visualize nothingness all around you and repeat ideas that make you feel happy. For example: "I am free from all earthly problems." "I feel no pain." "I am a good person." "I have nothing to fear." The more you repeat positive affirmations, the more you will believe the words you are repeating. Take a few quieting breaths and imagine your body slowly floating back to Earth. Picture yourself floating lower and lower: above the world, country, state, city, and building, until you visualize yourself back in your original position. As you open your eyes, you should feel a calm sense of peace come over you.

Relaxation Exercise #3

Sometimes you cannot do a lying-down relaxation exercise because you are at work or riding in a car. For these times, try the following exercise. First, close your eyes, take a deep breath, and hold it. Then tighten every muscle in your body as tight as you can. Take note of what it feels like to have every part of your body in a tense position. Hold the tension for a few seconds. Then open your mouth wide and exhale as long as you can from the back of your throat, making a loud hissing noise. As you exhale, relax your body and think of blowing all the tension in your body out through your mouth. Repeat this exercise two or three times. Then sit quietly and visualize your body free from tension and stress. Notice what it feels like to eliminate tension from your body.

Breathing Techniques

In today's busy world, we sometimes forget how to breathe! It is not uncommon for people who are in pain to take short, shallow breaths that deprive themselves of the oxygen they need. By breathing slowly and deeply and practicing healthy diaphragmatic breathing (rather than chest breathing), you can calm your entire body and help it function more efficiently.

It has been proven that experiencing certain feelings, such as pain, fear, or frustration, can change your breathing pattern. In these stressful states, you may breathe faster and retain carbon dioxide in your lungs. Over a short period of time, shallow breathing results in increased muscle tension and pain. It's a vicious cycle: pain causes bad breathing patterns and bad breathing patterns cause pain.

It's important to understand this cycle and be aware of your breathing. If you abandon bad breathing habits and remember that diaphragmatic breathing can be extremely relaxing to the autonomic nervous system, you will experience a calmer mind and relief from tightness in your muscles. Good breathing can ensure better blood flow through your body; your senses will heighten, and you will become more alert.

> **Fast Fact**
>
> People with fibromyalgia experience many symptoms that can be attributed to erratic breathing or hyperventilation (breathing too fast). These include …
>
> ◆ Dizziness
> ◆ Fainting
> ◆ Paresthesia (a tingling of the skin)
> ◆ Palpitations
> ◆ Chest pain
> ◆ Anxiety

How to Do Diaphragmatic Breathing

The diaphragm muscle should be the main muscle used for breathing. It is located at the bottom of your sternum (breast bone) in a part of the body that allows it to help your lungs expand and contract. Below it are soft organs that can move when a deep breath expands your rib cage outward. Above it are the lungs, which are also soft and pliable. In one breath, the diaphragm can move up and down as much as six inches. This movement can massage your lower organs and help return blood to the heart.

It is important to practice diaphragmatic breathing by doing the following:

1. Wear loose-fitting clothes and sit up tall in a chair with your feet flat on the ground.

2. Place your right hand on your stomach just over your navel.

3. Take a deep breath through your nose, feeling the air start to fill your body at your navel and moving up to fill your entire chest. You will notice that your hand moves as your stomach expands outward. You should hardly notice any movement in your chest or shoulders.*

4. As you slowly exhale, you will notice that your stomach deflates and your hand falls inward, back to its original position. The movement your hand is experiencing is the movement of your diaphragm.

5. Take a moment to rest and then repeat steps 3 and 4. If you start to feel dizzy, rest for 30 seconds and then proceed taking slower breaths.

   If you are noticing movement in your chest, put your left hand over your heart and concentrate on breathing from your diaphragm, which will ensure that your left hand is not moving.

It is important to practice good breathing seven to eight times a day, so that your body will eventually remember how to breathe properly.

Proper breathing can be achieved by practicing deep diaphragmatic breathing.

(Illustrations courtesy of Craig Kennedy.)

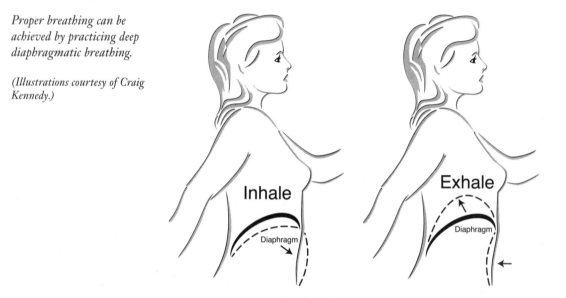

Developing Your Own Lifestyle Changes

Make a list of specific changes you want to institute in different areas of your life. After you have identified the changes, prioritize them so that you can establish a timetable to make those changes. There is room for your own Personal Plan for Lifestyle Changes in Appendix C at the end of this book.

The Least You Need to Know

- Change helps develop appropriate coping behavior, helps reduce stress, and restores a sense of order and purpose to our lives.

- Certain changes are necessary for you to adapt to a lifestyle that is healthier and will not inflame your symptoms.

- Individuals with fibromyalgia have a wide variety of problems associated with sleep.

- Research has found that when people with fibromyalgia reach a deep level of sleep, alpha brain waves intrude and jolt them back into shallow sleep.

- By setting a stable pattern for your sleep, you will help reset your biological clock.

- By breathing slowly and deeply, practicing healthy diaphragmatic breathing (rather than chest breathing), you can calm your entire body and help it function more efficiently.

Chapter 16

Healthy Lifestyle Changes: Exercise and Diet

In This Chapter

- ◆ Knowing the importance of exercise and diet
- ◆ Exercising with fibromyalgia
- ◆ Dieting for fibromyalgia
- ◆ Saving energy to reduce symptoms

After you have evaluated and made changes in your lifestyle to improve your quality of sleep, you need to address two more important aspects of your self-management plan: exercise and diet. This chapter explains how to make healthier lifestyle changes through exercise and diet.

Exercise

After a fibromyalgia diagnosis, one of the first things your health-care professional might suggest is to exercise on a semidaily basis. It would not be surprising if your first reaction was, "You have got to be kidding!" People with fibromyalgia experience pain with activity, so they naturally avoid exercise. Unfortunately, the result of less exercise is a deconditioned body.

Although recent studies have touted the benefits of exercise for helping people with fibromyalgia, each individual will have different kinds and levels of exercise that work best for him or her. Some health-care professionals feel that aerobic exercise is best, whereas others recommend starting with gentle stretching exercises.

When you are told to exercise, you might reflect back on your previous level of working out—running a couple of miles or spending an hour on the fitness machines at the gym. This may conjure up feelings of inadequacy and frustration because of your current decreased level of activity. It is important not to compare yourself to your previous standards or to others. You must find the boundaries that you can do *now* and accept these new boundaries. Do what is your personal best. Just like when you were healthy, a proper amount of exercise or, as you may want to refer to it, physical activity, will allow you to become more active and feel better as time goes on.

To find out what works best for you, you need to go through some trial and error. If you experience an increased amount of pain, you are probably doing too much. You do not want to do exercises that result in pain and exhaustion, causing you to end up in bed for several days. The idea is to do an exercise program that begins *very* gradually, allowing you to have very few, if any, negative side effects and ensuring that you can function the next day. You must remember that this is going to be a slow process and that you must be willing to set limits for yourself. It might be tempting to push yourself on a day when you feel good, but it is better to do too little than to do too much. The goal is to make your exercise program a positive experience.

Although the medical community has not come to agreement on any specific exercise program recommendations, the consensus seems to be to begin with very gentle stretching exercises and then work up to low-impact walking or swimming. A study published in the November-December 2007 *Journal of Clinical and Experimental Rheumatology* found that exercise therapy done three times a week for 16 weeks in a warm-water pool significantly reduced fibromyalgia pain as well as improved cognitive function.

Another safe way to strengthen your body is to use therapeutic bands or cables. These come in progressive resistances (yellow, green, red, blue, and purple). Check with the manufacturing company that makes the bands, so that you can start with the color that provides the least resistance and then slowly work up the color spectrum. One positive aspect to this kind of exercise is that it can be done at home. Eventually you might be able to work up to an aerobic program including cycling, running, or dancing. Some studies suggest that weight-bearing exercises are appropriate and beneficial for people with fibromyalgia.

Picture This/Lessons Learned

Picture This:

Because exercise is so important to your overall symptom reduction, it is important to find an enjoyable way to become physically active. If you previously enjoyed dancing, moving and gliding through warm water in a pool can give you the sensation of dance movements. If you used to like outdoor sports, go to the park to do your stretching exercises. And if competitive sports were your thing, set your own schedule to compete with yourself. Challenge yourself to work toward doing something that will help you to achieve a new standard of exercise, something that you have been unable to do since your diagnosis. Plan to walk a short distance in a local walk-a-thon, or swim a certain distance in a warm-water pool.

Lessons Learned:

Prior to having fibromyalgia I used to do a lot of bike riding. I found that a tandem bike was just the thing to get me back in the saddle. Instead of having to "go it on my own," the tandem bike gave me an opportunity to ride, but I didn't have to work as hard as I would on a single bike! The team approach allowed me the opportunity to exercise in a way that I truly enjoy.

You must listen to your body and let it tell you what it can handle. Again, each individual reacts differently to different types of exercise. The one thing that is important to keep in mind is that a deconditioned body continues to become weaker and weaker. Lack of exercise can cause tight, painful muscles; can reduce the functioning capacity of your cardiovascular system; and can cause weight gain. An exercise program that produces benefits must be developed specifically for you. It takes patience and persistence, but the results can be tremendous: decreased pain, increased flexibility, improved circulation, better sleep, relaxed, healthier muscles, decreased vulnerability to flare-ups, increased energy level, and a decrease in your level of anxiety.

Gentle Stretching

Stretching can start out as your main form of exercise and should always be done before and after low-impact and aerobic forms of exercise. Fibromyalgia pain causes muscles to shorten and tighten. A daily program of stretching helps warm the muscles by increasing blood flow and lengthening them, protecting you from the chance of injury. Breathing and relaxation exercises are excellent complements to a stretching program. As a form of exercise, stretching should be done for several minutes every day.

Healthy Alternative

Select a muscle group and then stretch the muscles for about three to five seconds, and then release. Then concentrate on mentally relaxing that muscle. Take a deep breath, exhale slowly, and begin the stretch again. This time you want to go further than the first time. You can hold the stretch for about 10 to 25 seconds. Remember to constantly breathe and mentally relax. Never bounce or force the stretch. If you still have questions, consult with your health-care professional or a physical therapist.

Low-Impact Exercise

After you feel comfortable with a stretching program, you will want to explore different types of low-impact exercises that appeal to you. In low-impact exercise, one foot should remain on the floor at all times, and you will be using the muscle groups in the lower part of the body. Along with the benefits of stretching, low-impact exercises also help improve joint flexibility and muscle strength and increase endorphins that promote a feeling of well-being. When you participate in a low-impact exercise class, such as a dance class or mall walking, you can eliminate isolation and increase socialization. If you experience an increase of your symptoms, you need to decrease the duration and intensity of your exercises.

Hydrotherapy—Warm Pool Exercises

Hydrotherapy is a form of exercise that takes place in a pool with a water temperature of at least 90 degrees. Warm-water exercise allows your muscles to relax and gives you the opportunity to move in a gravity-free environment that is less taxing on your joints and muscles. By using a flotation device while in the pool, you will remain upright while walking or moving through the water.

Dr. Daniel Rooks, at Beth Israel Deaconess Hospital in Boston, has developed an innovative approach for resolving problems associated with intense pain after performing land-based exercises. Dr. Rooks and colleagues performed a study that required patients with fibromyalgia to engage in four weeks of pool-based exercise. They then began a 16-week regimen of land-based exercises designed to increase muscle strength, cardiovascular endurance, and range of motion. Dr. Rooks and his colleagues anticipated that introducing low-impact, pool-based exercises first would help people with fibromyalgia experience fewer increases in pain when they began doing the land-based exercises. Dr. Rooks and colleagues also thought this would help eliminate emotional distress resulting from additional pain after exercise and encourage patients to continue exercising. In addition, the researchers anticipated that the water-based range-of-motion exercises would probably produce some increase in muscle strength that could be further enhanced during the land-based phase of the program.

Although Dr. Rooks and colleagues only studied 15 individuals, the results showed that the participants did display significant improvement in muscle strength and exercise tolerance, as well as in ratings of pain, fatigue, anxiety and depression, stiffness, and symptom interference with work. This suggests that using Dr. Rooks's innovative approach might help you minimize the initial increases in pain and anxiety associated with exercise.

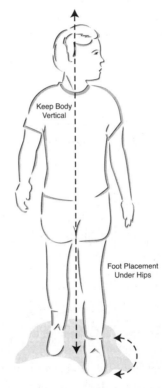

Keep Body
Vertical

Foot Placement
Under Hips

When walking heel-to-toe, make sure that your shoulders are back and that you are standing up straight.

(Illustration courtesy of Craig Kennedy.)

Daily Activities

Remember, all kinds of physical activity can be considered exercise. Walking your dog, gardening, strolling through your local shopping center, playing with your kids, or walking up and down your staircase several times a day can all keep you physically active. Remember to just keep moving!

Pain Signal

A word of warning: you must avoid activities involving sustained repetitive motions. Not only do these often cause repetitive motion injuries such as tendonitis and bursitis, they also tend to aggravate fibromyalgia pain, leaving you in pain that can be difficult to control.

Aerobic Exercise

Aerobic exercise is any activity that uses the large muscle groups and is maintained on a continuous basis. Aerobic activity causes the heart, lungs, and cardiovascular system to provide oxygen more quickly and efficiently to every part of your body. As the heart muscle becomes stronger and more efficient, a larger amount of blood can be pumped. By doing aerobic exercise, you can even trigger the body's own pain control system.

So how much aerobic exercise is recommended? Again, it varies from person to person. Most health-care professionals agree that you will benefit from 20 minutes of aerobic exercise three to four times a week. Because there are a variety of aerobic exercises to choose from, pick one that does not intensify your fibromyalgia symptoms and be very careful of impact injuries.

Following are some aerobic exercise options:

- ◆ Running
- ◆ Bicycling
- ◆ Fitness machines
- ◆ Jumping rope
- ◆ Skiing
- ◆ In-line skating

Healthy Alternative

Why does exercise help reduce symptoms?

Experts theorize that exercise changes the chemicals in the brain. It is thought that exercise provides both biological and psychological benefits that help people to feel better and improve their functioning.

Exercise Program and Rewards Chart

Here is a healthy way to start exercising. On a weekly basis, create a program of exercise that fits within your health boundaries. Remember, it is extremely important to listen to your body and not to push beyond your current level of comfort. Decide how much time you can tolerate and devote to that exercise program. Then on a daily basis, chart the exercises performed, the amount of time you dedicated to exercise, and how you felt after performing the exercises; reward yourself points on the following scale:

- Three points per day if you meet your goals

- Two points per day if you accomplished some of your goals

- One point if you recognized that your health won't allow you to exercise

- Zero points if you just skip your exercise program

Decide at the beginning of the week what your rewards will be depending on how many points you earn. Types of rewards might include having a massage, taking extra time for yourself to read, watching your favorite video, buying a CD or a pair of earrings that you have wanted, or starting a new hobby. At the end of the week, tally your points. If you have accumulated …

- 12 or more points, you can reward yourself the top reward.

- 8 to 11 points, you can reward yourself the runner-up reward.

- 7 or fewer, you get no reward. (If, however, you were not able to meet your goal because you were paying attention to what level of exercise you felt your body could tolerate … reward yourself for working within your limits!)

Here is an example of a possible exercise goal and how to chart your daily progress.

Sample Week 1 Goal

Type of Exercise	Amount of Exercise
Sitting on the floor slowly stretching the following body parts: neck, shoulders, arms, hands, back, hips, legs, feet, and toes.	Every day, for five minutes in the morning and afternoon.

Daily Progress Chart

Date	Exercise	Completed	Time	Results	Reward Points
6/6	Stretching		5 min.	Minor soreness	3
6/7	Stretching		5 min.	Mild fatigue	2
6/8	Stretching		5 min.	Very sore	3
6/9	Stretching		1 min.	Too sore	1
6/10	Stretching		5 min.	Felt good	2
6/11	Stretching		5 min.	Felt good	3
6/12	Stretching		None	Forgot	0
				Total Points:	14

Don't forget to reward yourself for all your efforts!

Tips for Conserving Personal Energy

Although this chapter has focused on exercising to improve your stamina and energy, sometimes your energy level will still be low. Energy levels in people with fibromyalgia can fluctuate from day to day. Each day, prioritize your tasks knowing that you might not be able to get everything done. The goal is to do more with less expenditure of energy. You can do hundreds of things to help preserve energy for the more important activities in your life. As you come up with your own ideas, add them to the following list:

♦ Many grocery stores now have prepared meals available to order, or you can order your groceries online and have the store deliver them to your home.

♦ Take a short rest two or three times a day, without going to sleep. Use pillows to prop yourself up and relax sore muscles.

♦ It is okay to ask your family for help. Create a list of tasks for everyone in the family so that dinner becomes a family event that won't wear you out. Assign yourself a task that won't involve lifting or standing for long periods of time. Then write down on small pieces of paper the other tasks that will be necessary to complete the meal. Have each member of the family draw one to find out what his or her task will be.

- If sitting is less painful and takes less energy, do tasks in a sitting position. Place pillows or blankets around you for comfort. Use a chair with wheels when available, so that you don't always have to get up and down.

- Be sure every telephone area or room in the house has a notepad, pen, scissors, important phone numbers, reading glasses, calculator, and other necessary items close at hand.

- Always place your keys and purse in the same place so you won't have to wander around looking for them.

- Always have a bottle of water with you when you go out. This helps with dehydration and ensures that you won't get thirsty.

- Keep a protein energy bar in your bag or purse at all times. If you feel hungry or light-headed, you will be prepared.

- Keep a folder of recipes for healthy meals that are quick and easy to make. Refer to these recipes to develop menu plans.

- Prepare several servings of casseroles, meatloaf, roast, or other dishes, so that you can eat one serving and freeze the rest for later in the week.

- Rearrange your kitchen so that the items you use most are in the most convenient places. If you need to get to pots and pans, there is no rule that says they always have to go on the bottom shelf. Create unique ways to store dishes and cups—such as stacking shelves or hanging racks that can be placed on your counter for easy access to get to them and put them away.

- Use rollout drawers installed in your cupboards (kitchen, bathroom, and so on) so you don't have to bend down and reach behind other items that are stored.

- When you go to the market, be sure that the clerk puts only a few items in each bag and do not hesitate to ask for help taking items to your car.

- Locate drive-up markets, cleaners, post offices, and pharmacies in your community, so you do not have to get out of the car when you are running certain errands.

- Give up something that you usually spend money on (soft drinks, fancy coffee drinks, cigarettes, having your nails done, your cable TV) and use the money for a housekeeper so that you can have your house cleaned once a month.

- Keep a small stepstool in your kitchen so you don't have to reach up to the higher shelves.

- Hang bathroom towels unfolded on the towel racks. Open the window so they will dry more quickly and will smell fresher; that way you won't have to wash them as often.

- Simplify your environment by decluttering your house. Keeping magazines, papers, trinkets, knickknacks, and general "stuff" around can clutter your environment and increase your time picking up and dusting.

- Consider using a slow cooker to prepare your meals throughout the day.

- Create lists before you go shopping. Plan exactly what route you will take to avoid traffic and to make sure that parking is accessible. Being prepared saves time and aggravation!

- Leave perfectionism behind. Learn how to prioritize the things that you want to spend your energy on.

- If you don't have the energy to organize or clean a specific room, close the door and know that you will get to it when you are feeling better.

- Serve food directly from the pan so you won't have as many dishes to wash. Designate a particular color glass to each family member and ask them to reuse it, so you won't have to do as many dishes.

- Have each family member take a turn planning the meals for the week.

- When standing, put one foot on a footstool to take the pressure off the small of your back.

Diet/Nutrition

When it comes to dietary and nutritional guidelines for people with fibromyalgia, again, there are a lot of differing opinions. It is apparent that additional studies are needed before we will know exactly what kind of diet is most beneficial. Until that time, many health-care professionals suggest following the Dietary Guidelines developed by the U.S. Department of Agriculture and adopted by the American Heart Association (AHA) for preventing heart disease. The basis for this diet is presented in the AHA's Food Pyramid, an outline of what to eat each day based on the Dietary Guidelines. The pyramid acts as a general guide that lets you choose a healthy diet from five different food groups. Although in recent years there have been discussions as to whether the original pyramid should be refined, in general most experts feel that eating healthy means consuming more fruits, fresh vegetables, beans, and whole grains.

Another diet that has recently received a great amount of attention and praise is the Mediterranean diet, based on dietary traditions of the people from the Mediterranean area (Crete, Greece, Southern Italy, and Northern Africa). Harvard University School of Public Health and Oldways Preservation & Exchange Trust developed the Mediterranean diet food pyramid in 1993. Although the two pyramids have several similarities, the difference is that the Mediterranean diet adds olive oil as a major food group—followed by cheese and yogurt, fish, poultry, eggs, sweets, and lastly red meat. According to the Center for Cardiovascular Education, "There is a general consensus among health professionals that the Mediterranean diet is healthier than the American diet because more grains, such as pasta and couscous, fruits, vegetables, legumes, nuts, and olive oil are consumed."

The popularity of the Atkins Diet, which restricts the amount of carbohydrates you consume, has raised the issue as to the benefits and risks such a diet produces. Studies continue to show that eating a well-rounded, balanced diet is, in the long run, easier to maintain and provides you with the overall nutrition that your body needs. It is thought that a balanced diet of both protein and carbohydrates will help maintain the right level of brain chemicals called neurotransmitters. These neurotransmitters carry impulses between nerve cells, and keep our moods under control by helping with sleep, calming anxiety, and relieving depression.

If you consume large amounts of carbohydrates, you can throw off your blood sugar levels. Carbohydrates tend to give you quick energy, but then as your blood sugar drops you can feel lethargic and moody.

Although the exact diet that people with fibromyalgia should eat still eludes us, we do know that by avoiding certain foods your general health will improve. Some feel that even fibromyalgia symptoms can improve. Substances you should avoid include foods with color additives and preservatives, aspartame, toxic chemicals, and high levels of fat. You should also avoid alcohol; cigarettes; caffeine-containing products such as coffee, tea, and chocolate; and products containing refined white sugar such as cakes and cookies. If you do decide to change your diet, remember to take it slow, making changes gradually over a four- to six-week period.

Food guide pyramid and
Mediterranean diet plan.

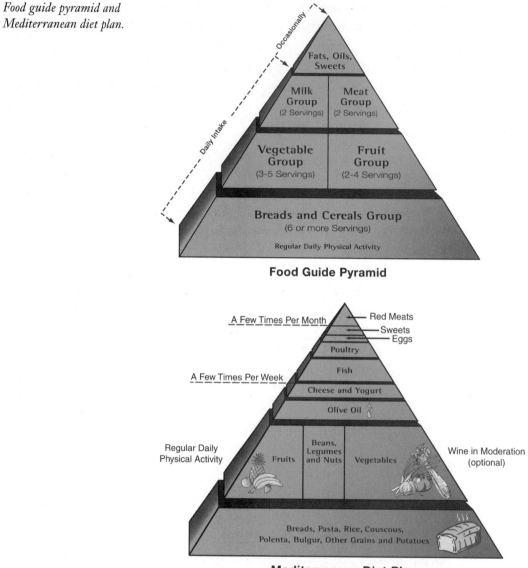

Food Guide Pyramid

Mediterranean Diet Plan

One way to help select healthy foods is by reading food labels. Today's labels can provide you with the following:

◆ Nutrition information about almost every food in the grocery store.

◆ Distinctive, easy-to-read formats that enable the consumer to quickly find the information they need to make healthy food choices.

◆ Information on the amount per serving of saturated fat, cholesterol, dietary fiber, and other nutrients of major health concerns.

◆ Nutrient reference values, expressed as % Daily Values, which help consumers see how a food fits into an overall daily diet.

◆ Uniform definitions for terms that describe a food's nutrient content—such as light, low-fat, and high-fiber—to ensure that such terms mean the same for any product on which they appear.

◆ Claims about the relationship between a nutrient or food and a disease or health-related condition, such as calcium and osteoporosis, and fat and cancer. These are helpful for people who are concerned about eating foods that may help keep them healthier longer.

◆ Standardized serving sizes that make nutritional comparisons of similar products easier.

Many people with fibromyalgia have overlapping conditions that require special diets. If you have been diagnosed with any of the following, take note of the dietary restrictions and suggestions.

Irritable Bowel Syndrome

It is estimated that between 50 and 75 percent of people who have fibromyalgia also have irritable bowel syndrome (IBS). IBS occurs in the large intestine and causes a group of symptoms including cramping, bloating, gas, diarrhea, and constipation. The nerves and muscles in the bowel are extra sensitive, and even eating a large meal can initiate symptoms and cause pain. People suffering with this syndrome may benefit by avoiding the following foods: fats, fructose (the simple sugar found in honey and fruits), milk products, chocolate, alcohol, caffeine, and carbonated soft drinks. A high-fiber diet may improve symptoms of diarrhea and constipation.

Lactose Intolerance

Lactose intolerance is the inability to digest lactose, the principal sugar of milk. This intolerance is caused by a shortage of the enzyme lactase, which is produced by the cells that line the small intestine. When there is not enough lactase to digest the amount of lactose consumed, a person may suffer from nausea, cramps, bloating, gas, and diarrhea. Individuals with lactose intolerance need to limit their intake of milk and dairy products or take lactase enzymes, which are available without a prescription.

Celiac Disease

It appears that small populations of people with fibromyalgia also have a digestive disorder called celiac disease (CD). CD is genetically predisposed and causes damage to the mucosal surface of the small intestine. This damage is the result of an immunologically toxic reaction to the ingestion of gluten. Gluten is a protein that is in all forms of wheat and related grains, rye, barley, triticale, and oats. CD can be diagnosed through a blood screening and a follow-up biopsy of the small intestine. People with CD must avoid eating all types of wheat and other noted grains.

Supplements

People with fibromyalgia should pay attention to general nutritional needs, because they often have absorption problems caused by digestive tract illnesses, such as bacterial overgrowth, celiac disease, and irritable bowel syndrome. Certain medications can also interfere with absorption, so adding nutritional supplements to your diet may be helpful. You do need to remember, though, that supplements are not a substitute for a healthy diet, and you must be cautious not to take too much of one nutrient because this can cause serious health problems.

The Food and Drug Administration (FDA) defines a supplement as vitamins, minerals, herbs or other botanicals, amino acids, and substances such as enzymes, organ tissues, glandulars, and metabolites. The supplement manufacturer is the one responsible for ensuring that its products are safe before it places them on the market. Drug products must be proven safe and effective for their intended use by the FDA before they are made available to the public; however, there are no provisions in the law for the FDA to approve dietary supplements. Therefore, you must be cautious. The challenge becomes finding out which vitamins and minerals you should take and which companies have the purest and most cost-effective products.

The best way to make these decisions is by talking to your health-care professional, a nutrition specialist, and the manufacturer of the product; by using your own common sense; and by doing some in-depth research. Although the Food and Drug Administration is not required to approve supplemental products, the more responsible companies do their own clinical research and have the results published in scientific journals. If you see claims that are unreasonable or sound too good to be true, such as "cures many diseases," or "all natural," be very cautious. Also beware of products that are backed by testimonials or have exorbitant prices. Just because a product claims to be natural does not mean that it is safe. These things should be considered when you make your supplement choices and compare one product against another.

An additional precaution that you can take is to look for the USP (United States Pharmacopeia) symbol found on some product labels. This symbol indicates that the product has met the USP standards for strength and purity. The mark assures consumers that a supplement has passed the following five quality tests under the USP's Dietary Supplement Verification Program:

- Contains the ingredients listed on the label.

- Has the declared amount and strength of ingredients.

- Will break down easily in stomach fluids so the body can effectively absorb the nutrients in the supplement.

- Has been screened for harmful contaminants such as heavy metals, microbes, and pesticides.

- Has been manufactured in safe, sanitary, and controlled conditions.

Some of the more common vitamins and minerals suggested for people with fibromyalgia include the following:

- B vitamins—Maintain healthy nerves, liver, help with energy production, and may reduce anxiety. Vitamin B_1 may support proper oxygen metabolism. The B-complex vitamins are essential to mental and emotional well-being.

- Calcium—Protects against bone loss. Low levels of calcium cause nervousness, apprehension, irritability, and numbness.

- Iron—Low levels can cause general weakness, exhaustion, and headaches.

- Magnesium—Provides for a healthy immune system and healthy nerves and helps with blood sugar regulation. Deficiency can cause confusion, apathy, and insomnia. Magnesium works well in conjunction with B-complex vitamins.

- Potassium—Depletion is frequently associated with depression, fearfulness, weakness, and fatigue.

- Vitamin D—In recent studies, 93 percent of people with musculoskeletal pain were found to be deficient in Vitamin D.

- Amino acids can also be helpful in promoting the healing process, and include the following:

  - Cystine
  - Glycine
  - Leucine
  - Lysine

- Valine

- Isoleucine

- Tryptophan and 5-hydroxytryptophan (5-HTP)—Helps to synthesize serotonin and melatonin

The FDA has posted safety warnings about the following:

- Dietary supplements that contain the herbal ingredient *comfrey*, which is a source of pyrrolizidine alkaloids. There is evidence that implicates these substances as carcinogens and that they may cause chronic liver disease.

- There have been reports of hepatic toxicity associated with products containing *kava*.

- Products containing *aristolochic acid*, including botanical products marketed as traditional Chinese medicines, have been associated with nephropathy—kidney disorder.

- The National Institutes of Health (NIH) showed a significant drug interaction between St. John's Wort (*hypericum perforatum*) and Indinavir and other antiretroviral agents.

- Dietary supplements that contain *tiratricol*, also known as triiodothyroacetic acid or TRIAC, a potent thyroid hormone, may cause serious health consequences, including heart attacks and strokes.

Overall, taking the proper precautions and discussing and informing your health-care team about the supplements you are taking can ensure safety and a positive outcome.

Obesity

Obesity is defined as too much fat in your body, which can cause a variety of health problems including high blood pressure, diabetes, heart disease, and stroke. In an Internet survey performed by the National Fibromyalgia Association and published in *BMC Musculoskeletal Disorders* in 2007, it was found that a majority of people with fibromyalgia tend to be moderately overweight, gaining approximately 35 pounds after developing the disorder. There are several theories on why people with fibromyalgia tend to gain weight, including inactivity, medications, and metabolic changes, but despite the reason, weight gain can cause both emotional and physical distress. Both exercise and diet play crucial roles in maintaining an appropriate weight. If you are overweight, weight loss can help reduce fibromyalgia symptoms and prevent you from developing other illnesses that can put your health at risk.

def•i•ni•tion

Body Mass Index (BMI) is a measure of your weight in relation to your height. It is the most widely used measure of a healthy weight. There is new evidence that supports the notion that being overweight tends to aggravate fibromyalgia symptoms, as well as predisposing you to develop diabetes. People with fibromyalgia who have diabetes tend to have more severe symptoms. To calculate your BMI go to: www.cdc.gov/nccdphp/dnpa/healthyweight/assessing/bmi/index.htm.

MEN		WOMEN	
Height	**Ideal Weight**	**Height**	**Ideal Weight**
4′ 6″	63-77 lbs.	4′ 6″	63-77 lbs.
4′ 7″	68–84 lbs.	4′ 7″	68–83 lbs.
4′ 8″	74–90 lbs.	4′ 8″	72–88 lbs.
4′ 9″	79–97 lbs	4′ 9″	77–94 lbs
4′ 10″	85–103 lbs.	4′ 10″	81–99 lbs.
4′ 11″	90–110 lbs.	4′ 11″	86–105 lbs.
5′ 0″	95–117 lbs.	5′ 0″	90–110 lbs.
5′ 1″	101–123 lbs.	5′ 1″	95–116 lbs.
5′ 2″	106–130 lbs.	5′ 2″	99–121 lbs.
5′ 3″	112–136 lbs.	5′ 3″	104–127 lbs.
5′ 4″	117–143 lbs.	5′ 4″	108–132 lbs.
5′ 5″	122–150 lbs.	5′ 5″	113–138 lbs.
5′ 6″	128–156 lbs.	5′ 6″	117–143 lbs.
5′ 7″	133–163 lbs.	5′ 7″	122–149 lbs.
5′ 8″	139–169 lbs.	5′ 8″	126–154 lbs.
5′ 9″	144–176 lbs.	5′ 9″	131–160 lbs.
5′ 10″	149–183 lbs.	5′ 10″	135–165 lbs.
5′ 11″	155–189 lbs.	5′ 11″	140–171 lbs.
6′ 0″	160–196 lbs.	6′ 0″	144–176 lbs.
6′ 1″	166–202 lbs.	6′ 1″	149–182 lbs.
6′ 2″	171–209 lbs.	6′ 2″	153–187 lbs.
6′ 3″	176–216 lbs.	6′ 3″	158–193 lbs.
6′ 4″	182–222 lbs.	6′ 4″	162–198 lbs.
6′ 5″	187–229 lbs.	6′ 5″	167–204 lbs.
6′ 6″	193–235 lbs.	6′ 6″	171–209 lbs.
6′ 7″	198–242 lbs.	6′ 7″	176–215 lbs.
6′ 8″	203–249 lbs.	6′ 8″	180–220 lbs.
6′ 9″	209–255 lbs.	6′ 9″	185–226 lbs.
6′ 10″	214–262 lbs.	6′ 10″	189–231 lbs.
6′ 11″	220–268 lbs.	6′ 11″	194–237 lbs.
7′ 0″	225–275 lbs.	7′ 0″	198–242 lbs.

Body Mass Index Chart.

The Least You Need to Know

◆ It is important to do an exercise program that begins very gradually, allowing you to have very few, if any, negative side effects and ensuring that you can function the next day.

◆ Some health-care professionals believe that aerobic exercise is best, whereas others recommend starting with gentle stretching exercises.

◆ Each individual reacts differently to different types of exercise.

◆ People with fibromyalgia should pay attention to general nutritional needs.

◆ If you do decide to change your diet, remember to take it slow, making changes gradually over a four- to six-week period.

Chapter 17

Dealing With Stress and Anxiety

In This Chapter

♦ Living in a stress-filled world

♦ Stressing over fibromyalgia

♦ Dealing with the symptoms of stress

♦ Recognizing depression

♦ Understanding the treatments for depression

♦ Taking back control of your life

When I first thought about my plight of having to live with a chronic illness, I began preparing myself for the worst—a life full of stress and anxiety. I thought that if I was constantly dealing with stressful symptoms, I was going to have to live in a state of constant uneasiness. I am pleased to share with you that this does not have to be the case! Despite your fibromyalgia, you can learn how to reduce stress in your life and how to deal with the anxieties that will confront you. But just as if you'd decided you want to become good at a particular sport or better at your job, it will take time and practice. You can, however, learn how to live a less stressful life, so that you can enjoy a healthier, happier existence.

This chapter will help you learn how to identify stressors in your life and ways to de-stress. You will also learn how to identify when you need help for medical conditions that have a psychological component, such as depression and anxiety. It is important to realize that stress can affect both your physical and emotional health.

Stress and Anxiety

It is hard to believe that we live in a time that is so technologically advanced, and yet 70 to 90 percent of the United States' population experiences high levels of stress on a daily basis. Our fast-paced culture causes us to feel anxious and uncertain about multiple aspects of our life. This stress causes wear and tear on our bodies. Unless we learn how to manage our stress, we will likely end up a society of sick and exhausted individuals.

You've probably heard people say things like, "I just can't seem to keep up with all there is to do!" Because we live in a society where there is so much opportunity, it can be exhausting trying to sort out what needs our attention and where to begin. Sometimes life feels like the volume has been turned up too loud or the weight of the world is on our shoulders—even if faced with just a small task. When life falls out of balance, for whatever reason, stress becomes a constant irritant, knocking things even more out of control.

In the case of fibromyalgia and other chronic illnesses, it is possible that the stresses in your life actually had an impact on your becoming sick. If you have a genetic pre-disposition to a certain illness, stress can act as an irritant and increase your chances of becoming ill. Think of it this way: if you have an open sore and you rub sand into the wound, the wound will get worse and it will not heal. In this analogy, the sand represents stress, and its role as an irritant will not let your body heal.

The reality is that chronic illnesses and the symptoms we experience often cause additional stress and anxiety, which make our pain and fatigue even worse. This is the ultimate catch-22, and the beginning of a terrible, vicious cycle.

Fight or Flight?

So why does stress have a negative effect on our bodies? Millions of years ago, the way the human body reacted to stress meant the difference between life and death. If a person was in a life-threatening situation, the body initiated the *fight-or-flight* response. To our ancient ancestors, the body's reaction to stress was based on a temporary situation. When the danger was over, their bodies returned to normal and they went back to their daily activities. Today, stress has a negative connotation. Instead of our bodies turning on the fight-or-flight response in dangerous situations, we are constantly reacting to aspects of our life that may be merely perceived threats.

def•i•ni•tion

Fight-or-flight is a biological response that releases endorphins, hormones, and glucose. Breathing becomes quicker, the heartbeat faster, and blood pressure higher. This gave our early ancestors the added strength to fight or flee the dangers surrounding them. This positive reaction to environmental circumstances was necessary for the preservation of the human species.

Our bodies also react to the multiple environmental stimuli that we are exposed to on a daily basis. As more and more opportunities are added to our lives, more stressors are also added. Today we don't need a threatening beast to walk into our camp to get our bodies revved up—all we need to do is wake up in the morning. Thinking about all the events of the day ahead, our body becomes instantly ready to fight or flee!

Picture This/Lessons Learned

Picture This:

You have fibromyalgia and you are sitting in your family room trying not to concentrate on your pain—but the TV is turned on to the evening news and the news anchor is talking about hundreds of people dying in the war. Your son and husband are having a conversation while playing with a handheld video game that makes an assortment of wild sounds. Your daughter is helping with dinner and the microwave timer is ringing, while at the same time she is using the blender to make her special salad dressing. And your dog is barking at the neighbor's dog, which is barking at the fire engine blaring its siren as it is going down your street. Your cell phone rings; it plays that annoying '60s song that you thought would be funny when you set up the ringer. You forgot to turn the cell phone off when you got home from the market and from picking up the kids at the soccer game after a nine-and-a-half hour day at work. Your boss "rewarded" you for doing such a great job by giving you an extra assignment that would take a "normal" person 50 hours. He knows that you will finish it in 10 hours, and of course you can't let him down because you are the number-one team player in the office and …

Lessons Learned:

Life is stressful. It is time for change.

The news, however, isn't all bad. Stress can have a positive impact, just as it did in ancient times. It can protect us and compel us into action. It can elevate our interest in new experiences and help give us a competitive edge. But if we overstimulate the body's senses or if we react intensely to situations where we have *feelings* of uncertainty, distrust, anger, and low levels of self-esteem, we will be constantly triggering negative physiological reactions.

By overwhelming our senses and allowing an intense level of emotional response to take place, we are overloading the body's response system, which will ultimately lead to health problems. To correct this situation, we must first learn to identify stressors that are not a real threat in our lives, and to react to them in a calm, balanced way. And second, we must better prioritize our lives and live within the goals we set to accomplish only what is reasonable. Stress will help or hinder us depending on how we react to it.

 Fast Fact _____

In times of stress, even a short reprieve from a stressor can make the situation less harmful to you both physically and emotionally. Try to remove yourself from the stressor and practice deep, slow, rhythmic breathing. Close your eyes and imagine a place where you feel safe and calm. In only a few minutes you will feel your body's reactions becoming more relaxed and the anxiousness caused by the stress will subside.

De-Stressing Improves Self-Esteem

One of the ways to deal with stress is to improve your opinion of yourself. A high level of self-esteem will help you to feel more in control, eliminating the need to feel uncomfortable or stressed in certain situations. The more comfortable you are in all aspects of your life, the less stressful you will find most situations. Self-esteem is the discrepancy between what you consciously think about yourself and what you want to be. The problem is that you might not be seeing yourself in a realistic manner or you might feel that your value is based on things that do not really matter.

For example, many of the things fibromyalgia patients attach to personal self-worth may no longer be possible for them to do. Your job might change or cease to exist, your purpose in life may now be different, you may become less independent, and your physical appearance may change. It is important that you view these changes with perspective. You are not your job. Everyone, even those who are chronically ill, has a purpose. You are not who you appear to be on the outside.

To eliminate stress and anxiety, it is important that you become comfortable with who you are in your new situation. If you always do your own personal best, whatever level that might be, you should feel the comfort of healthy self-esteem. Remember to keep your thoughts and actions in balance. The extremes in life are what cause stress and inner chaos.

Healthy Alternative
To help with your self-esteem, it is important to dialogue with yourself in a positive way. Every day, spend several minutes, morning and night, talking out loud to yourself, encouraging yourself, and congratulating yourself for the efforts and advances you have made. Even if you don't believe some of the things you are telling yourself, you will start to change your self-perception over time, and become more positive.
Here is an example of what you might say to yourself:
"Today was a good day. A neighbor came by to see how I was doing. I am worth visiting because I am an interesting and fun-loving individual. I was able to be of help to my neighbor. She was concerned because she had to make lunch for 12 Girl Scouts. I wanted to help because I am a caring individual, so I gave her my recipe for easy-to-make 'got-to-love-it chili.' She called me this evening to tell me that it was a hit and she wanted to thank me for being a good friend."

Identifying Stress Triggers

As with other health risks, each individual needs to recognize his or her own stressors. What might be stressful to one person might not be stressful to another. Things become stressful because of your reaction to them. If you pay attention to what situations, thoughts, and emotions bring on stress, you can identify them and avoid them, shorten your exposure to them, or change your response to them. If you are aware of the symptoms of stress, it will be easier to recognize the source of your stress.

This chapter points out that stress can be a positive thing. But only *you* can determine what level of stress is helpful and at what level it's destructive. There is no single level of stress that is optimal for all people. We are all individual creatures with unique requirements. Also, our personal stress requirements, and the amount of stress we can tolerate before it becomes dangerous, vary from person to person. Stress tolerance also changes with age. Obviously, the raging hormonal days of youth involved a different type of stress than the stress one may feel as a mother of three children, for example.

Many illnesses are affected by unrelieved stress. If you experience stress symptoms, you have gone beyond your optimal stress level; you need to reduce the stress in your life or improve your ability to manage it.

Physical and emotional symptoms of stress include the following:

- Irritability

- Inability to concentrate

- Sleeplessness

- Lack of or increased appetite

- Angry reactions to normal events

- Feelings of being out of control or overwhelmed

- Tension in your body, including your muscles

- Stomachaches

- Headaches

- Heart palpitations

- Nervousness and a feeling of panic

- Shaking or sweating

- Performing activities at an unusually rushed pace

- Feeling tired during the day and then using stimulants (coffee, sugar, chocolate) to help you keep going

- Using drugs or alcohol to help you calm down

- Being "tied up in knots"

Depending on how you react to a situation, almost anything can become a stressor! Walking into a crowded room, wondering whether you will ever feel better, hating life because you cannot understand why you have fibromyalgia can aggravate symptoms of stress you are already experiencing. It is important for you to identify the things in your life that cause *you* the most stress. Don't forget to identify various situations (such as seeing the dentist), thoughts (such as worries about finances), and emotions (your self-esteem) that can cause you stress.

After you become aware of the stressors in your life, you need to apply intervention strategies to reduce your stress. Many of the interventions you can apply are also helpful in managing the physical symptoms of fibromyalgia.

Ways to Relieve Stress

The following are ways to relieve stress that may be helpful for you to consider:

Change Your Lifestyle

- ◆ Improve sleep*
- ◆ Take time to exercise*
- ◆ Eat a healthy diet*
- ◆ Learn to relax*
- ◆ Increase leisure time
- ◆ Decrease stimulation in your environment
- ◆ Let go*—do not be afraid to cry

(*Refer to Chapter 15 for a more in-depth look.)

Change Your Thinking

- ◆ Think positively
- ◆ Improve your self-esteem
- ◆ Reframe your thinking
- ◆ Adopt more moderate views
- ◆ Refrain from trying to please everyone

Become More Organized

- ◆ Pace your activities
- ◆ Learn to say no when appropriate
- ◆ Keep a journal of thoughts and activities
- ◆ Prioritize your tasks
- ◆ Keep a realistic/healthy schedule

I Can't Be Depressed—I'm a Happy Person!

As stated previously, a diagnosis of fibromyalgia often comes after a long and exhaustive search for an explanation for your symptoms. You might see several health-care professionals, each one running multiple tests, but none of them providing any definitive answers. When your health-care professionals cannot come up with a diagnosis, you may think (or be made to feel by the doctor and the situation) that there is no physical basis for your complaints. It is no wonder that you may begin to think that you have "gone crazy." When you have not been offered any other explanation for your pain and fatigue, it is not unusual to jump to the conclusion that it is all in your head!

Fast Fact _____

Some of the neurochemicals in the brain that can affect mood are serotonin, norepinephrine, and dopamine. If these chemicals are out of balance, a person can feel uninterested in life and in things that were once important.

Today we know that fibromyalgia is a physiological condition; however, like any chronic illness, especially one that may take months or even years to get diagnosed, there are psychological aspects. Certain environmental situations or a genetic predisposition can lead to depression.

Depression is not simply feeling blue. It is a real chemical problem that develops into a medical illness with many physical symptoms, feelings, and thoughts that affect every aspect of your life. Although depression affects everyone to some degree at some point, only some people become medically depressed.

As Peter Farvolden, Ph.D., C.Psych., of the Depression Center in Toronto, Canada, notes, "... depression is not a sign of weakness. People with a depressive illness can't just 'pull themselves together' or 'tough it out' and get better. Without treatment, the symptoms of depressive disorders can last for months, even years. Fortunately, appropriate treatment can help most people with depression feel better."

The question, then, is what causes you to become depressed? Many people who find themselves diagnosed with both fibromyalgia and depression have never experienced depression before. It might come as a shock and result in feelings of embarrassment or guilt. The symptoms themselves may seem foreign, especially when you consider yourself a happy
person. It is important to know that depression is
an illness that _can be treated_ and usually very successfully.

One consequence of fibromyalgia can be depression. It can be brought on by one or more of these situations:

- An extended pre-diagnosis period

- Disrespectful or unsatisfactory medical treatment

- Personal grief and loss experienced as a result of having a chronic illness

- Lack of support from family, friends, and others

- Sleep deprivation

- Coexisting chronic health conditions

- Childbirth or menopause

- Lifestyle changes resulting from the inability to work or to carry on with your usual social, family, and other responsibilities

- The stress suffered by severe, continuous chronic pain

- Biochemical/neurotransmitter deficiencies (including serotonin, norepinephrine, and dopamine)

Because fibromyalgia has multiple symptoms, many of which are the same as depression, it's easy to miss the signs of depression. Sometimes the symptoms develop slowly over time and you may not be aware that you are experiencing them.

If you have lost interest in activities that used to bring you enjoyment or if you avoid participating in the normal activities of life because you feel empty, lonely, or fatigued, it is time to discuss your symptoms with a health-care professional. It may be uncomfortable admitting that you are depressed, but by denying it, you are denying yourself treatment. Because coexisting illnesses have a relationship to one another, by treating your depression, you should also see improvement in your fibromyalgia.

The following are some of the symptoms of depression:

Physical Symptoms (with No Medical Cause)

- Loss of appetite and weight loss; or overeating

- Digestive tract problems: nausea, stomach pain, constipation

- Sleep disturbances

- Decreased energy

- Difficulty with concentration and memory

- Headaches, muscle tension

Changes in Behavior

- Inability to make decisions or deal with small problems

- Restlessness and anxious behavior

- Avoidance of responsibilities

- Self-destructive behavior

- Irritability

Changes in Emotions

- Loss of enjoyment in activities previously enjoyed

- Feelings of sadness, pessimism, emptiness

- Excessive feelings of guilt, worthlessness, and helplessness

- Seeing life as overwhelming and out of control

- Loss of sexual desire

- Seeing life as hopeless and not worth living

- Thoughts of suicide

I had never experienced depression prior to having fibromyalgia, so I thought that only certain types of people became depressed. I have since learned that depression is not unique to any specific group of people. It is extremely common and can affect people of all ages, races, and levels of income and intelligence. It has nothing to do with being a positive person—and most importantly, it is nothing to feel ashamed of. Going through the necessary steps to get help may be unnerving or frightening, but the payoff—recovering the joy of life and feeling like yourself again—is well worth the effort.

The Depression Test

Dr. Farvolden developed the following Depression Test. This test is not designed to make a diagnosis of depression or take the place of a professional diagnosis. *If you suspect that you are depressed, please talk to your doctor as soon as possible.*

1. For the past two weeks or more, have you been feeling depressed, sad, or flat most of the time?
    ❏ Yes   ❏ No

2. For the past two weeks or more, have you lost interest or pleasure in things you usually enjoy?
   ❏ Yes ❏ No

3. Have you ever had a sudden period of intense fear, anxiety, or discomfort?
   ❏ Yes ❏ No

4. Are you anxious about going to or being in some places or situations because you …
   Fear that you will have an anxiety attack?
   Fear you will not be able to escape if you have an anxiety attack?
   Fear that help will not be there if you need it?
   Feel uncomfortable?
   ❏ Yes ❏ No

5. Do you avoid going to or being in some places or situations because you …
   Fear you will have an anxiety attack?
   Fear you will not be able to escape if you have an anxiety attack?
   Fear that help will not be there if you need it?
   Feel uncomfortable?
   ❏ Yes ❏ No

6. Do you have an excessive fear of, or do you avoid, social or work situations because you feel embarrassed, humiliated, or that people are judging you?
   ❏ Yes ❏ No

7. Do you experience anxiety because of uncontrollable thoughts, images, or impulses that you can't control?
   ❏ Yes ❏ No

8. Do you do certain things or repeat certain thoughts over and over again? Do you do these things according to special rules or until it feels just right? (For example, washing, ordering, checking, praying, counting, or repeating words.)
   ❏ Yes ❏ No

9. For the past six months or more have you been worrying constantly or excessively about several different things? (For example, work, school, family, finances, or health.)
   ❏ Yes ❏ No

10. Have you experienced or seen a traumatic or terrible event that included death or serious harm, or the threat of death or serious harm, to you or someone else? (For example, sexual assault, rape, accident, assault, disaster, war, or torture.)
    ❏ Yes   ❏ No

Total your responses: ____ Yes ____ No

Scoring: Total the number of yes and no answers you marked. If you marked yes five or more times, you may be depressed. You should consult with a health-care professional immediately. If you believe that you are experiencing symptoms of depression, talk to your health-care provider.

The Depression Center, Toronto, Canada: website: www.depressioncenter.net/; phone: 416-596-6715; e-mail: support@depressioncenter.net.

People experience depression differently and to varying degrees; therefore, each person responds uniquely to different types of treatment. Treatment often consists of counseling combined with medication. No matter what type of treatment you pursue, you need to take an active role in your treatment protocol. For example, it is important that you take your medication regularly, be honest with your health-care professional/counselor and yourself, and adopt healthy lifestyle habits including sleep, socialization, and diet. Because the support of your friends and family will be helpful, you should ask them to play a role in your treatment. It is important that you stick with treatment, even if it seems to be going slowly. We are very fortunate that today there are many pharmacological treatment options, and if one does not seem to help, there are always others that you can try.

Medications used to treat depression can take four to eight weeks before they are effective. Each medication works differently and on different neurochemicals. Because at this time there is no way to test which neurochemicals are out of balance, you and your health-care professional need to try different medications based on your symptoms. There can be side effects, so it is important you keep your health-care professional well informed. If you experience negative side effects, there are other options including increasing or decreasing the dose or even switching to a different medication.

Fast Fact _____

Referring to certain medications as antidepressants is not actually correct. This makes the patient think that the medication is used only to treat depression. The truth is that these medications are used to treat a range of symptoms including pain, sleep disturbances, and anxiety. It is important to talk to your physician about the reason he or she prescribed antidepressants.

If you are seeing a psychiatrist, it is likely that he will assist you with both your counseling and prescription medications. If, however, you are seeing a counselor who is not a medical health-care professional, your medication prescriptions will need to come from a medical health-care professional. It can be very helpful if your counselor or psychologist has a working relationship with your prescribing health-care professional. Ask your doctor to provide you with the names of health-care professionals that he or she works with. Make sure that your health-care team is communicating in order to coordinate your medical needs.

Who Should Treat Your Depression?

As stated earlier, depression is usually treated with counseling or medication. Counseling for depression may include the following:

◆ Cognitive behavior techniques

◆ Stress management skills

◆ Grief and loss issues

◆ Adjustment to chronic illness

◆ Anxiety management

◆ Support for difficult issues

◆ Counseling regarding a prolonged pre-diagnosis period

◆ Marital/family issues

◆ Working through past issues, such as sexual abuse

◆ Restoring hope

From the Fibromyalgia Assessment Clinic Patient Education Workbook, Abbott Northwestern Hospital.

When determining who will treat your depression, you have a variety of options. Because therapists specialize in different approaches (for instance, behavior modification, psychoanalysis, existentialism, or a humanistic approach) you should research these different styles or ask the opinion of your family health-care professional or rheumatologist. Prior to seeing a therapist, you need to understand his or her credentials. For a psychologist, look for a Ph.D. or Ed.D. (doctor of philosophy or doctor of education) or a Psy.D. (doctor of clinical psychology). For a psychiatrist, look for an

M.D. (medical doctor) or D.O. (doctor of osteopathy), with a residency in psychiatry. It is important to note that there is a group of psychiatrists who are not therapists and perform only medical evaluations.

Even finding a qualified practitioner does not always mean a perfect fit. If you do not feel comfortable with the health-care professional you have chosen, you should switch and find someone with whom you feel more comfortable. Remember, though, that you are not looking for a friend. You want a therapist who can be objective and forthright with you.

Taking Control of Your Circumstances

One of the easiest ways to feel in control of your life is by refusing to let difficult circumstances defeat you. Ironically, if you let go of preconceived notions, past mistakes, and trying to "do it all," you will let life be what it is—beautiful. We must face our own personal tragedies, and yet at the same time we must continue to pursue our dreams. Recognize that some things cannot be changed and put your energy toward those that can. In a world where you refuse to concentrate on your fears, you will find a life full of possibilities!

Feeding Your Soul

If fibromyalgia has left you feeling jaded and lacking enthusiasm for life, you have probably forgotten the importance of leaving your problems behind and scheduling some time for fun. It is easy to get into a monotonous routine—trying to just get through a day of pain. We forget an important ingredient in reducing stress and anxiety: doing the things that make us happy and fulfilled. Although we sometimes feel guilty about taking time for ourselves, it is an important aspect of living a healthy life.

Simple things can feed our soul and make us feel good. Here are some ideas to get you started:

♦ Add something beautiful to your day (for example, a bunch of flowers, a picture of a loved one, or a piece of art).

♦ Make sure you have quality time with the people you love.

♦ Notice things that are good about the day (for example, the good weather, or who you visited).

- Take time to practice your faith and recognize the power of your beliefs.

- Give yourself a hug and tell yourself what a good person you are.

- Always remember that you are more than your pain, more than your illness, more than your limitations. You have a body, mind, *and* soul. It is your soul that makes you unique and ensures that you have value and worth.

The Least You Need to Know

- In times of stress, even a short reprieve from the stressor can make a situation less harmful to you both physically and emotionally.

- Things become stressful because of your reaction to them. If you pay attention to which situations, thoughts, and emotions bring on stress, you can identify and avoid them, shorten your exposure to them, or change your response to them.

- After you become aware of the stressors in your life, learn how to apply intervention strategies to reduce your stress.

- Depression is not simply "feeling blue." It is a real chemical problem and medical illness with many physical symptoms, feelings, and thoughts that affect every aspect of your life.

- Treatment for depression usually consists of counseling combined with medication. Today there are many pharmacological treatment options for depression, and if one isn't helping, there are always others that you can try.

Chapter

Chasing Perfectionism

In This Chapter

- ◆ Noticing perfectionism in our society today
- ◆ Leaving perfectionism behind is important
- ◆ Learning about different types of perfectionists
- ◆ Discovering whether you are a perfectionist
- ◆ Knowing the health risks of perfectionism
- ◆ Discovering perfectionism traps

If you choose to live your life in pursuit of perfectionism, you will be putting your health in jeopardy. Perfection is not obtainable, so, by definition, you are setting standards that are unrealistic, resulting in personal frustration and stress. Those who strive for excellence in a healthy way understand that working to your own personal best is the most effective way to achieve great things. Perfectionists, on the other hand, are full of self-doubt and fears of rejection. When you are dealing with a disease that impacts your ability to function, it is important that you set realistic goals for yourself. If you work to achieve your best on that particular day, then you have set realistic standards for yourself and you will feel good about your accomplishments rather than disappointed.

Leaving Perfectionism Behind!

Those who consider themselves perfectionists are often proud to boast of their never-ending propensity to set unreasonably high standards for themselves—always overexerting, never knowing when they have done enough, and living in a constant state of stress. But what those striving for perfectionism don't realize is that their lifestyle can be both mentally and physically damaging. Wanting to be "perfect" is not a healthy pursuit of high standards, but rather a lifestyle that can cause debilitating emotional turmoil and feelings of worthlessness.

Perfection is humanly unattainable and indefinable. This chapter examines how you put your health at risk when you place yourself in a chronic state of stress as you strive for perfection.

The Myth of Perfectionism

If perfectionism is an unbalanced and unhealthy lifestyle, why are there so many of us who brag about being self-proclaimed perfectionists? The answer is easy. Society has led us to believe that perfectionism will provide us with positive outcomes. We are constantly exposed to media that tout the benefits of workaholism, claim that we "can have it all," flaunt visual images of what a truly perfect body is, and offer statements that influence us. They influence us to believe in the importance of striving for standards that aren't realistic. Many of us become duped into believing that if we push ourselves harder both mentally and physically then we will be rewarded with all that is right and good. Unfortunately, what we end up with is living life in a manner that leaves us frustrated, depressed, and sick. Perfectionism is not what it is touted to be!

Fast Fact

If you set goals for yourself that are not realistic, you will forever be chasing something that will remain elusive. If, however, you set goals that may take time and patience to reach, but are attainable, just think how incredible you will feel when you succeed! Remember your goals can change over time, because life is dynamic.

Instead we must not buy into the myth of perfectionism but rather focus on pursuing goals that are in balance with our own individual character and circumstances. We must focus on the goals that enable us to achieve our own high standards of excellence. Many people report a clearer perspective on life when they let go of unrealistic goals and learn to be proud of achieving their own personal best. If we try to establish our own standards based on other people's achievements, we will constantly feel that our achievements are never quite good enough. The feeling of self-accomplishment is rewarding and fulfilling. If we set standards that are unachievable, we will never experience the reward of self-accomplishment.

What Are the Signs of Being a Perfectionist?

Perfectionists come in all different types. There are those who feel that they have to do everything perfectly, and others who expect perfectionism from others. Then there are those who believe that others expect them to be perfect, and they are constantly trying to live up to standards that they think others have set for them. The main characteristic common among all these people is that they try to achieve standards that are unrealistic. These individuals believe their self-worth is based on their performance. Perfectionist thinking can start early in childhood, where these tendencies are actually attempts to find acceptance, approval, and love from others. Instead of working toward their own set of goals, they are constantly trying to meet and exceed the needs and standards of others. The more they try to figure out ways to please everyone else, the more they feel distressed and overwhelmed.

I am not quite sure when I moved from "doing my best" to wanting to do everything "perfectly." It might have been sometime during my high school years when I started to think that I would be more accepted and loved if I could just please everyone … my teachers, friends, those who were popular, my boyfriend, my parents, even strangers! No matter when you "cross over the line" and begin to strive for the unattainable, the sooner you can identify this unhealthy lifestyle, the better. Here is an opportunity for you to find out if you are a perfectionist.

Perfectionist's Test

Are you still living a life of perfectionism? Test your ability to set realistic goals that will help you to set standards that are appropriate for you.

Q: Is asking for help a sign of weakness?

A: *No. One way to get something done is to ask for help. Others like to be needed, and working together on a task can ensure a good outcome. A team process can be fun and very rewarding.*

Q: Is it important to never make mistakes in front of others?

A: *No. Making a mistake in front of others may be embarrassing, but it is not the end of the world. Actually, most people respond to a person's mistakes in a positive way because it makes the person more human. If you admit your mistakes, others often will respect you for your honesty and will admire you for your humility.*

Q: Should you never admit that you have made a mistake?

A: *No. Being truthful is a quality that most people admire. If you are willing to admit to a mistake, others will recognize your desire to correct the problem and learn from your mistakes.*

Q: Is there a right way to do things?

A: *No. For every problem, every situation, and every task there are millions of ways of accomplishing the same thing. Some may be better than others, but there is no one right way!*

Q: Is there always more that you can do to make something its very best?

A: *No. It is important to know how much time a certain project deserves. If you never finish something, then you never get to experience the satisfaction of being finished and knowing you have done the best you could. Remember the process is only part of the job—if you don't know when you are done then your efforts will never have a chance to be put to good use.*

Q: Do you have to feel stressed to make sure you are putting enough effort into a project?

A: *No. Stress is a response to a negative situation. Over time it can cause both emotional and physical health problems. Your goal should be to work in a calm, stress-free manner.*

Q: Should you avoid taking risks because you might fail?

A: *No. To achieve your personal best, you have to be willing to take some risks. Failure is a way to learn things, and accepting the fact that you will make mistakes is part of human nature.*

Q: Is being a workaholic a compulsive behavior?

A: *Yes. It is wonderful to have a job that you enjoy, but in order for you to live a balanced, healthy life it is important that you enjoy many other aspects of life besides just work. It is important to your general well-being to learn how to relax.*

Q: When you take on a task, should you always do it in an all-or-nothing way?

A: *No. There are things in your life that you will give your all, but not every aspect of your life has to be done to such an extreme. Give things the attention they deserve and know that you have done a good job if you have given your personal best.*

Q: Should you try something even if you are not very good at it?

A: *Yes. No one is good at everything, and it can be fun and challenging to try something new. You will become a more diverse and interesting person if you try things that are new and unfamiliar to you. This is especially important if you can't do something you used to do well—it can be an adventure finding new things that you can do now that might not have interested you in the past.*

Q: It is reasonable to be preoccupied with the fear of failure?

A: *No. Fear can keep you from doing something that might be reasonable. Ask yourself if you are afraid of something that others aren't afraid of. If your answer is yes, then you might have an unrealistic fear caused by the fear of failure. These are the fears that you want to overcome so they won't keep you from experiencing important aspects of life.*

Q: Is it true that a mistake means that you are unworthy?

A: *No. A mistake means you made a mistake this time.*

Q: Are all goals hard to achieve?

A: *No. Goals can be challenging, but if you set realistic goals for yourself, you should be able to eventually accomplish your goals and then move on to the next set of realistic goals you have set for yourself.*

Q: Does saying "no" to a project or task mean that you are cowardly?

A: *No. Learning to say no can be very healthy. If you are saying no because the situation compromises your health, makes you do something against your ethics, allows you to express the truth, or allows you to avoid a situation that you do not feel comfortable in, or to protect your family—then by all means say no!*

Placing Your Health at Risk

One of the most important reasons you should leave your perfectionist tendencies behind is because of the toll they can take on your health. If you are living with a chronic illness, the last thing you want to do is practice a lifestyle that puts even more stress on your body. If you are constantly trying to live up to unrealistic expectations, you are putting your body under constant stress—stress that can exacerbate any existing health condition(s).

When your body reacts to stress, the nervous system is activated along with specific stress hormones. Hormones such as adrenaline and cortisol are released into the bloodstream. Your heart and breathing rates speed up and your blood pressure rises. These physiological changes prepare the body to act quickly in an emergency situation. These changes can protect you in a short-term situation, but when they become a part of your daily experience they can have a negative effect on every system in your body. The end result can be a depleted immune system, leaving you exhausted and at-risk for infections. Many of the hormones that can disrupt the nervous system can also affect your digestive track. This can cause diarrhea, constipation, bloating, and an increase in digestive acids. Studies have also shown that stress can intensify pain, especially in the muscles of the shoulders, neck, back, and face. And the adverse health effects don't stop there. Prolonged stress can also have an impact on your mental health. If you are constantly worrying about attaining certain levels of perfection, the disappointments you will experience can turn into anxiety, anger, and frustration. If you are constantly worrying, you will suffer concentration gaps and lapses in your memory. In the long run, if your expectations are constantly unmet, you can even become prone to depression. Without time to relax and enjoy the lighter side of life, your unhealthy ways will weigh you down, leaving you vulnerable to a host of emotional disorders.

Pain Signal

Avoid:

Fatigue

Loneliness

Absoluteness

Rigidness

Extremes

Stressors

Seek and Find:

Breath

Acceptance

Laughter

Alleviation

Nurturing

Confidence

Exercise

The Perfect Trap

When I first found out that I had fibromyalgia, I vowed to do everything I could to get better, and I wanted it to happen *now*, not later. I would set timelines for getting better. I could "afford" a month of being sick, but that was all I could accept. Then each time one of my self-imposed deadlines for getting better wasn't met, I would sink deeper into feelings of desperation and frustration. Every time a new symptom appeared or an old one reappeared, I would endlessly analyze everything I did prior to the pain and fatigue. I approached my illness like I had always approached other aspects of my life. I was going to fight, fight, fight! Struggle, struggle, struggle!

I was obsessively focused on finding the answers to get better. I wasn't going to be weak and ask for help, I wasn't going to say no to things even if I knew that they weren't healthy for me. I was not going to let anything change! I was not about to expect anything less than perfection from myself in this task. No matter how I was feeling, I was going to remain in control. I kept running away from the reality of my situation. Like I said, I believed nothing was going to change!

It is ironic how a person can want something so much and think that they are doing all the right things to accomplish it, only to wake up to a totally new reality. I don't mean I gave in to it, but rather that I listened to my body and started to set reasonable expectations for practicing a self-management plan. My compulsive analysis of everything did nothing but make me more anxious, and I had to practice patience over time. By asking for help, others felt they could contribute something positive to the situation, bringing us closer together and encouraging mutual compassion and better communication.

I found that life was much less complicated when I set realistic priorities and realized that all I had to do was give my best effort. Reasonable efforts produced positive results. I put my mistakes behind me and instead of focusing on what could have been, I focused on what would be. And by facing the future with a positive attitude, I felt a power over my situation that I had never felt before. I learned that it was totally ridiculous to expect myself to "please everyone." By letting go of that expectation, I experienced a freedom that I had never experienced before. It was an incredible feeling that came from realizing the value of doing a few things well, rather than many things not so well. The fear of change eventually became absurd to me.

Change can be an exciting and rewarding occurrence. The biggest and best change that I experienced was learning that imperfect results do not lead to catastrophic consequences. And as I set realistic goals, more of my goals were met and life became much more pleasurable. Life is not black or white and neither is having fibromyalgia. If you can avoid all-or-nothing thinking, you'll find a life full of opportunity and new ways to create a more tranquil journey.

The Least You Need to Know

- Perfection is humanly unattainable and indefinable. So by choosing to strive for something that is always going to place you in a chronic state of stress, you will also be putting your health at major risk.

- Society has falsely led people to believe that perfectionism will provide them with positive outcomes.

- Focusing on pursuing goals that are in balance with your own individual character and circumstances will enable you to achieve your own high standards of excellence.

- If you are living with a chronic illness, the last thing you want to do is practice a lifestyle that puts even more stress on your body.

- If you are constantly trying to live up to unrealistic expectations, then you are putting your body under constant stress, which can exacerbate any existing health condition(s).

- With time you will learn that the way to find control over your illness is to let go and learn how to accept it.

Chapter 19

Finding Support Groups and Organizations

In This Chapter

◆ Knowing the benefits of a support system

◆ Understanding what makes a good support group

◆ Finding a support group

◆ Evaluating a support group facilitator

◆ Attending a support group can be beneficial for your family

Wherever you are in the process of dealing with fibromyalgia, there are others out there feeling just like you. In fact, local and national organizations can put you in touch with others who know exactly what you are going through. Your fellow patients can prevent you from feeling alone, provide you with credible, up-to-date information, and help you connect with resources that are truly helpful. This chapter shows you how to find the support you need.

Finding Support in Others

When you suffer from an invisible disease (one where you don't look sick), it can be comforting to have the understanding and support of others who share the same challenges you are facing. Instead of getting a blank stare when you talk about your symptoms, others who have fibromyalgia will react with genuine understanding because they have lived through similar experiences. Most people want to know that what they experience is normal. If you talk to someone who has "been in your shoes," your feelings will be validated and you'll know that someone understands you and cares about you.

Fast Fact _____

The fibromyalgia community is served by a national patient advocacy organization that is headquartered in Anaheim, California. For assistance contact them at:

National Fibromyalgia Association
2121 S. Towne Centre Place, Suite 300
Anaheim, CA 92806
714-921-0150
www.FMaware.org

Support Group Directory: www.fmaware.org/site/PageServer?pagename=community_supportGroupDirectory

The National Fibromyalgia Association has a newsletter for support group leaders called the *FAME Support Connection*. This monthly online newsletter provides information and assistance to support group leaders across the United States. Go to www.fmaware.org/site/PageServer?pagename=community_fameSupportConnectionNewsletter.

What Is a Support Group?

A support group is a group of people who gather together because they share a similar situation, problem, or illness. The goal of the group is to offer support and share information that helps provide education, resources, and solutions to the issues group members are dealing with. The activities of the group are determined by the needs of the participants.

Most fibromyalgia support groups are independent, local groups that are organized by volunteers. Some groups are associated with hospitals or individual doctor's offices. Often the group's facilitator is self-appointed, so it is extremely important that you investigate a group's beliefs and "personality" before embracing what it has to say. Support groups can vary in many ways, and it is important for you to make sure that the group or groups you attend are organized in a way that will be beneficial to you.

During your research into community groups, you will find that some groups are very informal and others are formal. An informal group involves a group-sharing situation where the general atmosphere is one of mutual trust. Formal groups consist of a moderator and a guest lecturer. No matter how a group is organized or which structure it establishes, it is most important that the focus is a positive one in which you learn how to deal with your illness—not focus on the negatives.

When looking for a local support group, you need to be sure that it meets the following requirements:

◆ Its focus is on providing you with *positive* information of an educational nature—it's not just people sitting around complaining.

◆ Its members discuss a wide variety of treatment options and do not push one particular product or method.

◆ You feel comfortable with the members of the group.

◆ The group is well organized and not dominated by one or two people.

◆ You have an opportunity to ask questions.

◆ It has a medical advisor or advisors to ensure that the information it is providing is accurate.

◆ The group is a continuing source of support.

◆ The group offers encouragement and promotes self-help and self-sufficiency.

◆ The group meets in a location that is convenient for you.

◆ When you leave the meeting, you feel better than when you got there.

Where do you go to find a local support group? Here are some ideas:

◆ National organizations often have a directory of local support groups and can provide you with contact information. Many of the organizations that can help you are listed in the back of this book.

◆ Many local groups have a website that provides information about the group and its meeting schedule.

◆ Hospitals, health-care professionals, libraries, health-food stores, and other local community groups that are interested in helping people often are aware of local fibromyalgia support groups.

◆ Your local newspaper may have a calendar or special section where it lists support group meetings. Look to see if they list a meeting time for people interested in fibromyalgia.

◆ Some support groups are associated with a church and may be listed in the church bulletin.

Support Group Members Contact List

The following is a list of information that you should collect about potential support groups and national organizations. Remember that you might be able to get help from groups that aren't just focused on fibromyalgia. For example, there may be support groups in your area that can help you with issues related to depression, anxiety, weight loss, financial issues, marriage counseling, and other areas that might also be affecting you. Always ask if the group provides resource lists or other information that can help you with ways to better manage your illness. Fill in this list of information when doing your research:

Support group contact information: _____

Group name: _____

Contact person: _____

Organization's purpose: _____

Meeting topics/speakers: _____

Meeting dates and times: _____

Meeting location: _____

Phone number(s): _____

E-mail: _____

Notes: _____

_____

_____

Healthy Alternative

When you are a member of a support group, you must ensure that the facilitator is doing their job correctly. Ask yourself if the facilitator does any of the following. (The answer to each question should be "Yes!")

Does the facilitator:

◆ Guide the discussions in a positive way?

◆ Provide a comfortable setting and allow for stretch breaks?

◆ Set a tone of sharing so everyone has a chance to contribute?

◆ Listen to what each member is saying?

◆ Enforce a confidentiality rule?

◆ Promote problem solving and encourage the group to help one another?

◆ Provide a well-rounded schedule of activities and topics?

◆ Thank the members for their contributions and acknowledge those who have volunteered their time to help the group?

◆ Ensure that information is accurate and unbiased?

Support Groups over the Internet

Meeting with support group members in person not only adds an element of social interaction to your life, but it can also encourage you to get out of the house and become less isolated. However, there are times when people with fibromyalgia are not physically able to get to a support group meeting in their community. During these times, you can "meet" with others in an Internet chat room or share thoughts and ideas on a subject message board. Just as you do when attending an in-person support group, always be sure that the information that is being shared is positive and accurate.

Fast Fact _____

The following groups have responsible and helpful chat rooms:

Immune Support.com: www.immunesupport.com/chat/fibromyalgia-chat.cfm

WebMD: www.webmd.com/community/all-boards

Yahoo! Groups: groups.yahoo.com/search?query=fibromyalgia

How to Win the Support of Family and Friends

It can be challenging for family and friends to understand your illness because they can't see it. Your pain is not obvious to them. Because fibromyalgia symptoms wax and wane, some days you are able to accomplish more than others—and that can be hard for your loved ones to understand, too. It's important for them to learn about fibromyalgia so they can support you as you deal with the illness. Therefore, you will need to make every effort you can to help educate and communicate the reality of your situation to those who are part of your life.

Explain to your friends and family that your symptoms are not imagined or easily overcome. Be truthful with them about when you are feeling bad—and when you are feeling good. Help them to understand why you sometimes may have to cancel plans you had both been looking forward to. And be sure to support your loved ones, too, with the challenges they are facing in dealing with your diagnosis. You should all be working together toward the same goal: to help you get better.

Share with the people in your life credible information that explains the reality of your situation. Books, magazines, or online articles from medical journals can help clarify the information you have been sharing with them. An excellent place to get this information is from national and local groups that have up-to-date information meant to be shared with family members.

Fast Fact _____

At most fibromyalgia support group meetings, only about 15 to 20 percent of the participants are spouses or other family members. If you encourage your family to attend a meeting with you, they will learn valuable information to help them better understand your situation.

Your "invisible" illness is going to have an impact on the people in your life—especially your immediate family. *Together* you need to understand what it means to have fibromyalgia—that it is no one's fault, and that by working together to deal with the problems and create solutions, everyone will benefit in the future.

It can also be beneficial if another party can help your family become objective and supportive. You may want to set up a meeting with your spouse or significant other and the healthcare professional who works with you to manage fibromyalgia, or invite your partner to a support group meeting. Family and marital counseling may also be helpful.

For some family members, it is easier to ignore the problem, because then they do not have to deal with it. But just as you do, your family needs to accept the situation for what it is right now, and find ways to communicate and work together to improve things for everyone. Often your family will benefit in multiple ways by attending a support group meeting with you. They can learn about what you are experiencing, as well as discover ways they can help themselves.

The Least You Need to Know

- Whatever the state of your condition, there are others who feel just like you do.

- A support group is a group of people who gather together because they share a similar situation, problem, or illness.

- No matter how a group is organized or what structure it establishes, it is most important that the focus is a positive one in which you learn how to deal with your illness—not focus on the negatives.

- Family can become educated about fibromyalgia by meeting with their loved one's healthcare professional, attending a support group meeting, or going to family and marital counseling sessions.

Twenty-Five Quick and Easy Tips for Feeling Better

In This Chapter

◆ Learning 25 different tips for feeling better

◆ Proving that small actions can have big rewards

◆ Finding heath-care tips that are easy and fun

◆ Using home remedies that really work

◆ Exercising more than one approach for better health

When we deal with a big problem, we often feel that it will take a big solution to help resolve the problem. Luckily, this is not always the case. Many difficult symptoms of fibromyalgia can be dealt with via small lifestyle changes or easy, unsophisticated treatments. It is always exciting to find a simple remedy that has a big effect on your health. Although some simple remedies have no steadfast scientific explanation as to *why* they work, we accept them because they *do* work. How many of us have suffered with a common cold, only to feel better after eating a bowl of Grandma's home-made chicken soup?

You should rest assured that like Grandma's soup, there are some easy tips you can practice to help improve fibromyalgia symptoms. Don't underestimate the impact that an easy tip might have on your quality of life!

Problems with Cognition and Memory

Tip: Slow down the pace of your life.

Explanation: Among the more common fibromyalgia symptoms are cognition and memory problems, affectionately referred to as fibro fog. Many memory problems result from doing too many things at one time or continuing to function even when you are overly fatigued. Slowing down and paying attention to the amount of thoughts and activities you are processing through your brain at one time can help reduce the symptoms of foggy memory. After you have reduced the amount of information you are processing, practice the following: repeat things to yourself, write things down, and eliminate things in your environment (noise, interruptions, excessive light, bad smells, and so on) that distract or overstimulate you. If you have to do something that requires a lot of concentration, try doing it at a time when you feel less fatigued.

Do the Things You Enjoy!

Tip: Find new things that you can enjoy despite your fibromyalgia.

Explanation: Sometimes we can't do all the things that we used to do because of our fibromyalgia, but that doesn't mean there aren't new things that you can do that will enrich your life! I found that I no longer had the stamina for dancing, something I had always loved doing, but I could move like I was dancing when I was in a warm-water pool. The enjoyment I experience when I "dance" in a pool is different from "land dancing," but it too can be wonderful!

Avoid Flares

Tip: Sometimes finding shortcuts around the house can mean the difference between having a productive day instead of an overtaxing day that leaves you exhausted and in pain.

Explanation: Take the time to think about the way you are doing household chores so you can recognize whether you are "working smart." Look at each task and write down the steps you take when doing the dishes, making the bed, or preparing dinner. If you are taking extra steps to complete the task, rethink your routine and eliminate needless steps.

Neck and Shoulder Pain

Tip: Never carry bags or purses over your shoulder. Use roller carts or cases that are easy to maneuver and won't weigh you down.

Explanation: Carrying heavy items on your shoulders can increase your chances of developing muscle pain and stiffness, as well as general fatigue. The use of a wheeled cart or briefcase can transport necessities without the burden of lifting and carrying items.

Sore, Stiff Muscles

Tip: Soak in an herbal bath and lightly massage your muscles with an herb-filled washcloth.

Explanation: A warm- or hot-water bath, filled with a mixture of soothing herbs, can calm sore muscles and relax your mind. Deep, moist heat can even calm your internal organs.

Take a small handful of each: valerian, lavender, linden, chamomile, hops, and burdock root; simmer the herbs for 15 minutes in two gallons of water. Strain the herbs from the infused water and place them in a soft cotton washcloth. Pour the infused water into your bath, adding enough warm water to fill the tub three quarters of the way full. Soak in the herbal water for 20 to 30 minutes. (If you have dry skin, reduce the amount of time you spend in the water.) Use the herb-filled cloth to lightly massage areas of your skin or muscles that are particularly painful or tense.

> **Healthy Alternative**
>
> While you are relaxing in your herbal bath, you might want to listen to music, meditate, surround yourself with candlelight, or just enjoy the quiet and calm.

Feelings of Stress, Loneliness, and Fear

Tip: Adopt a pet.

Explanation: Research shows that pets have a therapeutic effect on their owners. They can actually reduce a person's blood pressure, muscle tension, and other physical stress responses. They also have a positive effect on their owner's mood. Animals are excellent companions who give unconditional love and don't talk back. They bring out our nurturing spirit and help us feel more secure and safe. Studies have shown that pet owners live longer, healthier lives. So what kind of pet is best? Pick a pet that fits your interests, temperament, lifestyle, and environment. Anything from a tropical fish, dog, bunny rabbit, or even a horse will have that effect; a pet has the ability to divert your attention away from your pain and beyond yourself.

> ### Healthy Alternative
>
> Having your own pet might be too much responsibility, but there is an alternative. Therapy Dogs International, Inc.'s (www.tdi-dog.org) primary objective is to provide comfort and companionship by sharing dogs with patients in hospitals, nursing homes, and wherever else therapy dogs are needed. Their goal is to promote healing and improve emotional well-being through the companionship and joy that can be experienced when a dog comes to visit!

Excessive Pain While Trying to Do Household Chores

Tip: Pay attention to your back. Household chores can put extra strain on your spine and the muscles in your back.

Explanation: Fibromyalgia pain can be exacerbated by simply doing the normal daily activities of caring for your home. To protect yourself from hurting your back or causing additional body strain, remember to practice the following:

- When you attempt to pick up a heavy object, always bend from the knees, not the waist. As you lift, hold the item as close to your body as possible. Turn by stepping in the direction you want to go. This will protect you from twisting your body and straining your spine. Think about what you are doing to prevent quick, painful movements.

- While talking on the phone, do not cradle the phone between your ear and shoulder. Always hold the phone with your hand, or better yet, use the speakerphone or a headset.

- Relax your back by taking rest breaks when doing household chores. If you sit on a couch, do not prop yourself up by using the couch's arm. This can cause your back to be put in an unnatural position and result in lack of circulation to your arms, shoulders, and back. Use smaller pillows at the small of your back or under your arms to provide you with support and good posture.

- When doing a chore that requires you to stand in one place for an extended period of time, use a footstool to prop up one foot. This takes the strain off your back and keeps you from locking your knees under you.

- Store pots, pans, and bowls in cabinets that are at waist level. This eliminates the need to bend and lift these heavy objects.

- Eliminate reaching and bending by using long-handled dusters, mops, and cleaning brushes. Use a "grabber-device" to help pick up lightweight items or things out of your easy reach.

- Share the chores with your family. This allows you to perform the tasks that are less stressful on your back and body.

- When doing laundry, don't overload a laundry basket and carry it through your house or down your stairs. Instead, place a few clothes in a dirty towel or sheet. Make the bundle light enough to carry or drag the bundle behind you. There is no need to carry laundry down a staircase when you can drop it over a railing.

Abdominal Bloating and Discomfort

Tip: Avoid certain foods.

Explanation: Some abdominal bloating and discomfort can be caused by intestinal sensitivity due to irritable bowel syndrome. One way to reduce these symptoms is to avoid certain foods. Suggested foods to avoid include the following:

- Broccoli
- Baked beans
- Cabbage
- Caffeinated drinks
- Carbonated drinks

- Cauliflower
- Chewing gum
- Fried foods
- Hard candy
- Nuts

Feelings of Stress and Anxiety

Tip: Have a good laugh.

Explanation: Humor is a wonderful stress reducer. A good laugh can relax tense muscles, help increase your oxygen intake, and help lower your blood pressure. When something makes you laugh, it gives you a different perspective on your problems. If you can laugh at a situation, it is no longer threatening or out of your control. So when you enjoy something humorous, you will physically and mentally reduce the symptoms of stress and anxiety.

Fast Fact _____

Humor is clinically proven to be effective in combating stress. Lee Berk, M.D., Ph.D., has demonstrated that laughter can prevent many physiological effects of distress. When you laugh, you lower your cortisol levels, which can help protect your immune system. For more information about Dr. Berk, see science.box.sk/newsread.php?newsid=4104.

Repetitive Strain/Stress Injuries (RSI) to the Hands and Arms

Tip: Adopt healthy computer practices to avoid RSI.

Explanation: You might experience pain in your hands or wrists after a long day at the computer or doing repetitive tasks. You can avoid aggravating wrist positions by adopting the following practices:

◆ Do not bend your wrists to the side. Rather, keep your fingers in a straight line with your forearm. Do not rest your wrists on the desk.

◆ Instead of hunching toward the monitor to read and straining your eyes and back muscles in the process, increase the font size on your monitor.

◆ Use a light touch on the keyboard. Also avoid gripping or squeezing the mouse.

◆ Use both hands to perform double-key operations to avoid twisting one hand to hit both keys.

- Take a lot of short breaks to stretch and relax. Pace and plan your computer work to allow time to exercise your neck, shoulders, hands, and back.

- Sit straight and do not lean forward to reach the keyboard.

- Adjust keyboard height so that your forearms are parallel to the floor.

- Keep your arms and hands warm. Cold muscles and tendons are more fragile and at a much greater risk for overuse injuries.

- Adjust your chair height so that your thighs are parallel to the floor.

How to Prevent Fibro Flares After Surgery

Tip: Make special arrangements with your surgeon and anesthesiologist.

Explanation: Robert Bennett, M.D. (www.myalgia.com), suggests that prior to surgery, you discuss your situation with your health-care professional and request and do the following:

- The arm with the intravenous line is kept near your body, not away from your body or over your head.

- Wear a soft neck collar and minimize neck hyperextension (especially if an endotracheal tube is anticipated).

- Be given a preoperative opioid pain medication about 90 minutes prior to surgery. Opioids are morphine or morphine-related drugs. The rationale for the preoperative use of opioids is to minimize central sensitization, which can worsen the widespread body pain that you are already experiencing.

- Have a long-acting local anesthetic infiltrated into your incision even though you will be asleep during the procedure. The rationale for this is to minimize pain impulses reaching the spinal cord and brain, which in turn drive central sensitization.

Most people with fibromyalgia require a longer duration of postoperative convalescence, including physical therapy in many cases. Some patients experience higher levels of pain and require a longer duration of postoperative pain medication.

Anxiety About Making the Right Decisions

Tip: Trust yourself.

Explanation: When faced with multiple decisions in a short period of time, you might question whether you are making the right decisions. If you pay attention to your thoughts and feelings, and act on what you think is right, you will make decisions that are right for you. Become educated about the pros and cons of an issue, and then act based on what makes you happy or falls into your comfort range. Others may give you their opinion, but ultimately the decision is yours and you must feel comfortable with it and the resulting outcome. Learn to listen to what your body is telling you and use that information to help make health-related decisions.

Facial and Jaw Pain

Tip: Protect your face and jawbone from excessive use.

Explanation: If you experience facial and jaw pain, it might just be part of your fibromyalgia symptoms or it might be temporomandibular joint disorder (TMJ). Alert your health-care professional to the symptoms you experience. To help reduce facial and jaw pain, do the following:

- Pay attention to the position of your mouth. Keep your lips almost together, but be sure there is no tension in the facial muscles. Do not clench your teeth together. Let the jawbone rest comfortably.

- When eating, try to limit the extent to which you open your mouth. Cut your food into very small pieces and chew with your back teeth. Do not bite into food with your front teeth.

- Until the pain subsides, try to eat foods that do not require a lot of chewing. Avoid chewing gum.

- Practice your relaxation exercises. With your eyes closed, breathe in through your nose, directing the breath to the areas that hurt. Then exhale, breathing out your tension and pain.

- Try sleeping on your back. Avoid placing the sides of your face on a pillow or mattress, because it might put pressure on your jaw.

- Rest is an important aspect of eliminating jaw pain. Try to get a good night's sleep; it helps in the healing process.

Migraine Headaches

Tip: Avoid certain foods and environmental situations that can trigger migraine headaches.

Explanation: There are many types of triggers for migraine headaches: bright or flashing lights, certain smells or exposure to toxins, exhaustion, hormonal changes, changes in the weather, stress, and so on.

A migraine headache can also be triggered by the foods you eat. Here are examples of the foods that are thought to trigger a migraine:

- Chocolate
- Aged cheese (especially cheddar)
- Eggs
- Alcoholic beverages (especially ones containing sulfites)
- Caffeinated beverages (at times caffeine can be helpful in reducing a migraine and might be an ingredient in a migraine medication you are taking)
- Citrus fruits
- Nuts
- Preservatives, sweeteners, flavor enhancers, monosodium glutamate
- Onions
- Cabbage
- Tomatoes
- Salt

Feelings of Guilt and Insecurity

Tip: Learn to be more honest and direct with yourself and your family, friends, and co-workers. Learn how to communicate.

Explanation: Living with a chronic illness can cause feelings of guilt and insecurity. Often, with the right communication, you can eliminate many of the negative feelings you experience.

Clearly communicate your thoughts and ideas to reduce misunderstandings and potential frustrations. Let others know how you are feeling and why you have to do things the way you do. Do not complain, but rather provide them with the information they may be lacking to understand your circumstances. Recognize that not everyone will be sympathetic or understanding, but as long as you have attempted to communicate with them, you can eliminate any guilty feelings.

 Pain Signal

Try to find a level of cooperation rather than attempt to change the minds of those around you. It is healthier to maintain an acceptance of each other's perspectives, rather than constantly debating over certain issues. By turning obstacles into opportunities and negatives into positives, you will experience less stress and remain calmer. Make practical suggestions rather than just restating the problem. Be sure that your suggestions are in the interests of all parties.

By making your feelings and needs known, you increase your self-esteem. Stand up for yourself firmly, but not aggressively. Practice "positive self-talk" to eliminate negative symptoms of stress. For example, try saying to yourself, "I am a calm, relaxed, and confident person."

Feeling Overwhelmed and Exhausted

Tip: Track your activities for one week, and then identify what activities are time wasters. Next create a strategy to eliminate or deal with each time waster.

Explanation: Throughout the day, some activities are not productive or take priority over more important activities. By identifying these time wasters, you can come up with ways to ensure that they are not making you feel overwhelmed or exhausted.

Obvious time wasters include the following:

- **Interruptions.** Establish a schedule that includes time when you are not to be disturbed. Make sure that your family and co-workers respect your time.

- **Inefficient meetings.** Ensure that there is a pre-established agenda and that the meeting participants keep to the outline. If you are only involved with part of the agenda items, arrange to only attend the meeting during that time.

- **Phone tag.** Suggest a specific time when a call can be made or returned. This allows both parties to be available and ready for the conversation.

◆ **Overcommitting.** Before you agree to do something or attend an event, seriously consider whether you have the time and interest. Do not feel guilty for saying no.

◆ **An impossible schedule.** If you set a schedule that becomes impossible to keep, prioritize your activities and eliminate those things that are less important or unnecessary. Recognize realistically how long it takes to perform each task.

◆ **Disorganized activity.** If you have several things to do in the kitchen, group those activities together and do them at once without straying to other projects in other areas of the house. Every time you stop and restart an activity, it takes additional time to get back into the flow of that activity.

◆ **Failure to think ahead.** If you are sitting down to read a book, first think about the things you will need. Make one effort to find the book, your glasses, a pillow, a footstool, and a drink. Then when you start reading you will not have to stop to get the things you need and want.

◆ **Disorganization.** Designate a place where you always keep your glasses, keys, purse, shopping list, address book, and so on. This will greatly reduce the time you spend looking for these items.

Sore Feet, Bruises, and Stomach Upset

Tip: Using earthy solutions can relieve pain, fatigue, and a variety of other symptoms.

Explanation: Earthy solutions include plants, herbs, and natural food products that can bring relief to health problems. Remember, however, that just because something is derived from a plant or is called natural does not mean that it is always safe. Use common sense and always tell your health-care professional what you are taking.

Examples of earthy solutions include the following:

◆ **Sore feet.** Soak sore feet in peppermint and chamomile tea.

◆ **Bruises.** Rub in Arnica oil or cream. Arnica Montana is a daisy-like mountain flower that seems to relieve bruising and swollen joints and muscles.

◆ **Intestinal upset.** Acidophilus changes the intestinal flora and reduces the chance of getting diarrhea, stomachaches, gas, and bloating.

◆ **Stomach upset.** Chamomile tea (made from the chamomile flower) can help relieve nausea and menstrual cramps, and promote sleep.

♦ **Cut or insect bite.** Lemon oil can act as an antibacterial antiseptic for minor cuts and insect bites. Lemon juice is a digestive stimulant that helps with digestion and constipation.

♦ **Anxiety.** Lavender tea possesses the ability to calm the nervous system and relax your mood. Even the smell of lavender can have a calming effect.

Picture This/Lessons Learned

Picture This:

If you are in bed and want to get up, here is a good four-step process to help you:

1. Lie on your back.
2. Place your right leg over your left leg and your right arm over your chest. This will help you to easily roll over onto your left side.
3. Roll more to the left, placing your forearms and elbows on the bed (or floor) and then slowly push yourself up so you are resting on your hands.
4. If you are on a bed, slowly swing your legs over the side until you are completely sitting up. If you are on the floor, tuck your legs up under your body and then use your hands to help push yourself up on your knees. Stabilize yourself by holding on to a table, chair, or person, before you place one leg at a time under you so you can stand up.

Lesson Learned:

If you take the time to move slowly and properly, you will protect yourself from unnecessary muscle strain and fibromyalgia pain.

Getting Out of a Chair Without Hurting Yourself or Causing Strain

Tip: Be sure that you use the following six-step process to get out of a chair to help protect yourself from muscle strains or joint pain.

Explanation: Follow these steps.

1. Place your hands on the front edge of the chair seat, on the outside of each of your legs.
2. Move your bottom close to the edge of the chair.

3. Place the ball of your right foot on the ground. Be sure that your foot is directly under your knee, forming your leg into a right angle.

4. Place your left foot flat on the ground about 6 to 10 inches away from the edge of the chair.

5. Push off with your right foot and your hands, rocking forward so that your weight ends up on your left foot.

6. If you are less stable, use the arms of the chair, a walker, or a person to help stabilize your movements.

Dry, Itchy Skin

Tip: Take steps to hydrate your skin and your body.

Explanation: Dry skin can be the result of a natural lack of moisture in the skin; an autoimmune disease, such as Sjögren's syndrome; eczema; system-wide dehydration; sun exposure; weather changes; or allergies.

To help prevent dry, itchy skin, implement the following dry-skin repair program:

◆ Drink at least eight glasses of water per day.

◆ Add vitamin E to your diet. Vitamin E is a fat-soluble oil that is found in vegetable oils, nuts, and green leafy vegetables. The recommended adult dietary allowance is 10 to 15 milligrams per day. Taken internally or by placing a small amount of the oil on your skin, it can help heal skin and scar tissue.

◆ Hot water can dry the skin. Avoid soaking in baths filled with soaps or perfumed products, which can also be drying to the skin.

◆ When you get out of the bath or shower, do not towel off completely. Leave some moisture on the skin and then apply a good dry skin moisturizing lotion or ointment. This will seal in more moisture to the skin. Aquaphor ointment is especially effective for very dry skin.

◆ For itchy skin, fill the bathtub with warm water and add colloidal oatmeal. Place some of the oatmeal in a cotton cloth, tied with a rubber band. Washing with the oatmeal will reduce itching.

Aloe vera gel is also very useful in relieving itchy spots. You can break off a stem from an aloe vera plant and rub the sticky insides of the plant on your skin, or you can purchase aloe vera in liquid or gel form at your local health-food store.

◆ Good circulation is also helpful for healthy skin. Inverted yoga poses, in which your feet are above your head, can help increase circulation and reduce toxins from settling into your lower extremities. Massage can also help improve circulation, and the masseuse can use oils to help combat dry skin.

Aches and Pains While Sitting at a Desk

Tip: Take breaks from work and complete a series of relaxation exercises that you can do at your desk.

Explanation: Depending on how you feel, you should take at least one short break per hour. Although it is not always possible to get up from your desk to take a break, there are things you can do *at your desk* that will help you feel calmer and experience less pain.

Slowly raise your shoulders in a circular motion, up to your ears and back down. Do this about 10 times, circling forward first and then reversing the motion to the back. If you still feel tense, shrug your shoulders up to your ears and hold this position. As you release your shoulders back down, breathe out and imagine releasing all the tension you are holding in your neck and shoulder muscles.

Sit back and close your eyes. Computers, bright fluorescent lights, and heavy reading can strain your eyes. Give them a break. You may want to use eye drops to help prevent dryness. After you have rested your eyes for a few moments, rub the palms of your hands together really fast until they get hot and then place your palms over your closed eyes. This will also help relieve eyestrain.

Put your hands out in front of you, wiggle your fingers, and shake your wrists for at least 30 seconds. You may want to also stretch your arms up over your head and stretch your spine upward toward the ceiling.

Take a deep breath in through your nose, hold it for a few seconds, and then breathe out through your nose. Repeat this five or six times.

Take your shoes off and, while sitting, stretch your legs out in front of you. Wiggle your toes, rotate your ankles in both directions, and then stretch your legs out in front of you as far as you can. Let your legs drop down to the floor and then repeat three times.

Give yourself a little massage. If your arms or feet are particularly sore, gently massage the area that is painful. If you are in a lot of pain, take time to apply ice to the sore areas. Using a frozen bag of vegetables can be a convenient way to do this.

Before you go back to work, check your posture, making sure that you are sitting up straight and breathing deep, refreshing breaths.

Mood Swings and a General Sense of Ill Health

Tip: *Aromatherapy* has been used for years to promote well-being and balance.

Explanation: Aromatherapy can be defined as the art and science of utilizing naturally extracted aromatic essences from plants to balance, harmonize, and promote the health of the body, mind, and spirit. It is a *noninvasive* treatment, designed to affect the whole person by using essential oils to promote the body's natural ability to balance, regulate, heal, and maintain itself. In aromatherapy, the oils can be massaged into your skin or you may just smell the oil for a short period of time. It is recommended that you consult with a qualified aromatherapy practitioner.

> **def•i•ni•tion**
>
> **Aromatherapy** is the use of extracts or essences from flowers, herbs, and trees that have been turned into oils and then are rubbed into the skin or breathed in through the nose to promote health and well-being.

Examples of essential oils include the following:

- **Clary sage.** Natural painkiller, helpful in treating muscular aches and pains. Very relaxing, and can help with insomnia and in balancing hormones.

- **Rosemary.** Very stimulating and uplifting, good to help mental stimulation as well as to stimulate the immune system. Very good for muscle aches and tension.

- **Cinnamon.** Antiviral antiseptic, promotes circulation, aids in digestion, and acts as a respiratory stimulant.

- **Dill herb.** Relieves indigestion, constipation, nervousness, gastric upsets, and headaches.

- **Frankincense.** This tree bark is helpful for fevers, coughs, colds, bronchitis, and laryngitis.

- **Jasmine.** The jasmine flower helps with depression, menstrual problems, and lethargy.

> **Pain Signal**
>
> Aromatherapy is not intended to replace traditional medicine or traditional health care. It is considered a complementary therapy to help ease symptoms.

Burning and Tingling Pain

Tip: Avoid activities and clothes that can accentuate the symptoms of burning, numbness, and tingling pain in the arms, hands, legs, and feet.

Explanation: With fibromyalgia your sensitivity to touch and temperature can cause symptoms that include weakness, numbness, burning, and abnormal sensations in the skin. There are several ways to avoid these irritating symptoms:

- ◆ Avoid wearing clothes that are constricting.

- ◆ Select clothes and sheets made out of fibers that are not rough to the touch.

- ◆ Avoid materials that don't breathe, and that retain moisture and perspiration.

- ◆ Always wear sunscreen and a protective hat.

- ◆ Don't leave your hands, arms, and legs in one position rubbing against a hard or rough surface. This can cause the skin to burn and tingle.

- ◆ Remove labels from clothes, so they won't become irritants.

- ◆ Exercise a small amount every day to increase your circulation.

- ◆ Avoid exposure to long periods of heat or cold.

- ◆ Take vitamins shown to reduce symptoms: B_1, B_{12}, and folic acid.

- ◆ Take supplements that have been shown to reduce burning and tingling, including magnesium, alpha-lipoic acid (also known as thioctic acid), and gamma-linolenic acid (GLA).

Sore, Aching Muscles

Tip: Draw toxins out of your body that might be causing pain and fatigue.

Explanation: Four great ways to draw toxins out of your body include the following:

- ◆ Get a body massage. Make sure that you drink a lot of water before and after the massage to flush out toxins.

- ◆ Take a steam bath. After the steam bath, be sure that you use cool water to wash off completely. Again, drink lots of water to flush your system.

◆ Use a wet loofah or soft body brush to gently wash and stimulate areas where your lymph glands are close to the skin (such as under your arms, neck, and groin area).

◆ Place one to two cups of Epsom salts in a warm bath and soak for several minutes. Epsom salts are known for their ability to help relieve sore muscles.

Runny Nose and Watery Eyes Due to Allergies

Tip: Eliminate dust, pests, and pollens from your bedroom by using an air filtration system and humidifier.

Explanation: Bedrooms are notorious for collecting dust, bed mites, cat and dog dander, and other allergy irritants. Because you spend a great deal of time in this room, it is important to use an air filtration unit. If you also experience dry skin, eyes, and mouth, you may want to add a humidifier. Make sure that you change the filters often and help the process by vacuuming under your bed, shaking and airing out mattress pads, and keeping pets off your bed.

Tension Headache

Tip: Check your body language. Are your muscles tense from holding your body in an unnatural way? If yes, adjust and release the way you hold your body.

Explanation: When in pain or under stress, you might find yourself curling up into a fetal position. You might hold your body out of alignment trying to "protect" the part of your body that is in pain. Often, pain causes you to roll your shoulders forward and pull your arms in around yourself, like an animal trying to protect himself. If you experience tension in your neck and shoulders, you might look like your shoulders are up around your ears. Another sign of tension is the pursing of your lips or clenching of your hands. If you are in pain, it might feel natural to draw inward or tighten your muscles to protect yourself from more pain. The problem is that this can actually elevate the amount of pain you are feeling. This kind of tension can even affect blood circulation to various parts of your body. One of the most common problems that arises from physical tension is a tension headache. Be aware of your body language and immediately relax into a more suitable position at the first sign of awkward body language.

The Least You Need to Know

◆ Even the simplest of things can have a positive impact on how you feel and function.

◆ Be open to new ideas and ways that might help reduce your negativity and symptoms.

◆ Fibromyalgia can be affected by even minor environmental changes. Learn how to care for yourself by monitoring, and if necessary, changing your environment.

Part  5

What Will the Future Be Like?

There are times when life with fibromyalgia will seem overwhelming and uncertain. The fact that this illness can wax and wane might cause you to wonder if the future will continue to challenge you with cycles of symptoms. Improvements may not come as quickly as you would like, and the disease may test your ability to stay strong and hopeful. Despite your temptation to feel despondent, you can rest assured that we are now moving forward in our understanding of the causes of fibromyalgia and we continue to have new and improved treatments. Research is expanding and more and more people are becoming interested in finding the answers to questions that will provide patients with new options. Specific medications have been approved to treat fibromyalgia and a new momentum to find additional pharmacological treatments has begun. We are living in a time that has more hope than ever before. It is important for you to surround yourself with people who are optimistic and know that new ideas and new treatments will become a part of your future.

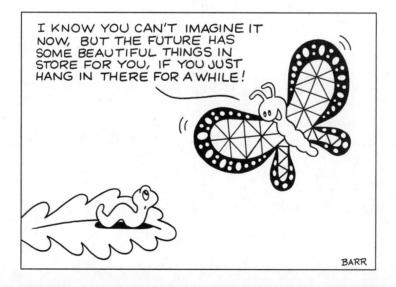

21

When Is Disability Appropriate?

In This Chapter

- Understanding Social Security disability
- Qualifying and applying for Social Security disability
- Understanding the role of an attorney
- Understanding the role of your physician
- Winning your case
- Getting back to work

In a survey conducted by the National Fibromyalgia Association in 2003, 99 percent of the respondents who were currently disabled because of fibromyalgia said that they would return to work immediately if they could find some relief for their pain. In my experience, people with fibromyalgia only apply for Social Security disability as a last resort—when it has become impossible for them to maintain work on a consistent basis. The reality, however, is that the disability process is a taxing one, and for someone with fibromyalgia it can be arduous at best. Many find the process too exasperating and give up only to find themselves living a financial nightmare.

In the majority of fibromyalgia cases, the individual can continue to work, but in some situations disability is not a choice but rather a necessity. In this chapter, you learn about being aware of your options, to seek help and advice, and to understand that disability does not have to be a permanent situation.

You Aren't Lazy

One of the most outrageous myths about people with fibromyalgia is that they are lazy. In truth, most people with fibromyalgia lead extremely active, productive lives both before and after their diagnosis. There are, however, those who are not able to work during certain stages of their illness and a few people who are not ever able to return to work. The thought of having to cut back or stop working even for a little while can be depressing and frustrating. Applying for disability goes against the desire to be self-sufficient, even when chronic pain and fatigue have made it impossible to remain in the workforce. Deciding to stop working to concentrate on improving your health is a very difficult one and should not be made without a great amount of thought and consideration.

It is important to note that the Social Security Administration has determined that fibromyalgia "can constitute medically determinable impairments within the meaning of the statute." Or in other words, a person with fibromyalgia can be found disabled if it is proven that they meet the accepted medical standards for disability. Social Security Disability Insurance is just that—insurance coverage for wage earners who have worked at least 5 years out of the last 10 years before they became unable to work. While you were employed, you were required to pay federal withholding and self-employment taxes. Each year, workers receive a summary of these contributions. Unfortunately, spouses in family businesses may be left out altogether if a separate contribution is not made. For those who do pay, however, the Social Security Administration must provide you with disability insurance benefits if you qualify under the federal guidelines (see Social Security online at www.ssa.gov/disability). The key here is that you have to prove that you are qualified.

> **Healthy Alternative**
>
> If you are concerned about being able to work, first consider trying these options: cut back the number of hours you work, get permission to work from home, talk to your employer about setting up an area where you can lie down and rest during the day, work the hours of the day that you usually feel best, or if necessary, find a different job that is not as stressful, not as demanding, or closer to home.

Social Security Disability Insurance

Several kinds of disability programs exist, including state worker's compensation, private pension disability, and public pension plans. The focus in this chapter is on Social Security Disability Insurance (SSDI), the model for all disability plans.

To be eligible for SSDI, you must be between the ages of 21½ and 65 and have worked 5 out of the last 10 years during the period before you became disabled at age 30. If you did not work at least 5 years in the past 10 years, even if you worked full-time in the years before that, you will *not* qualify for SSDI unless you are less than 30 years old.

Social Security disability benefits range between $350 and $1,800 per month, and access to Medicare begins after 24 months of benefit payments. The 5-month waiting period is not included in the 24 months. It is important to remember that the payment of benefits can be 12 months before the date of application plus the 5 months of the waiting period.

If you think this is complicated, it is. The onset of disease is usually not the onset of disability. To qualify, you have to meet Social Security's qualifications, which are determined by five questions:

1. Are you working?

   If you are working and your earnings average more than $800 a month, you cannot be considered for disability. However, this is not a hard-and-fast rule and there are exceptions.

2. Is your condition "severe"?

   Your condition must interfere with basic work-related activities for your claim to be considered disabling.

3. Is your condition found in the list of disabling impairments, and if not is it sufficiently severe?

   The listing is contained in the booklet "Disability Evaluation Under Social Security." The Office of Medical Evaluation is the source of all Social Security information pertaining to medical issues. Here is the address to obtain a copy of the booklet.

   Office of Medical Evaluation
   Office of Disability
   SSA 6401 Security Boulevard
   Baltimore, MD 21235

The list of disabling impairments is maintained by Social Security. Certain impairments are considered so severe, that they automatically qualify you as disabled. Fibromyalgia is not on the list, and must be decided based upon medical and vocational (or work-related) considerations. Those rules are not easy to find because they take concepts from a wide body of regulations, case law, and vocational evidence.

4. Can you do the work you did in the last 15 years?

If your condition is severe, but not at the same or equal severity as impairment on the list, it must be determined whether it interferes with your ability to do the work you did in the last 15 years. If it does not, your claim may be denied. There are rules that incorporate age, education, and past work experience, which may affect the entire situation.

Fast Fact _____

Studies such as the occupational environmental study by George Waylonis, M.D., are useful in looking at the types of work activities that cause problems for people with fibromyalgia.

5. Can you do other work?

If you cannot do the work you did in the past, you will be evaluated to see whether you are able to adjust to other work. To be disabled you must be unable to perform an unskilled, sit-down job on a full-time, regular basis. If you cannot adjust to other work, your claim will be approved.

The Definition of Disability

It is important to understand how Social Security defines disability. Each disability program has its own definition for disability. Some programs pay for partial or short-term disability benefits. Social Security does not. Disability under Social Security is based on your inability to work. It is all or nothing. You will be considered disabled if you cannot do your past, relevant work and the SSA decides that you cannot adjust to other work because of your medical conditions, your age, and your education. Your disability also must last or be expected to last for at least 12 months.

The SSA categorizes musculoskeletal impairment as "Regardless of the cause(s) of a musculoskeletal impairment, functional loss for purposes of these listings is defined as the inability to ambulate effectively on a sustained basis for any reason, including pain associated with the underlying musculoskeletal impairment, or the inability to perform fine and gross movements effectively on a sustained basis for any reason, including pain associated with the underlying musculoskeletal impairment. The inability to ambulate effectively or the inability to perform fine and gross movements effectively must have lasted, or be expected to last, for at least 12 months."

How and to Whom Do I Apply?

As soon as you know that you are not capable of working any time in the next 12 months and that you have a valid disability case, you should contact the Social Security Administration (the SSA nationwide number is 1-800-772-1213) and request an application to apply for disability. You can also visit the website at www.ssa.gov for electronic filing. If the connection should fail before the application is completed, take a deep breath and try again.

Pain Signal

When applying for disability, you are placing yourself in a stressful situation. Be prepared to feel frustrated and exhausted by the process. If you recognize that this is going to be a long, difficult course at the beginning, you can mentally and physically prepare yourself for the ordeal.

Prepare to answer the following questions when you first apply for SSDI:

Your name at birth and now

Birth date and location

Your gender

Social Security number

If you or anyone else has ever applied for you to receive Social Security benefits, Medicare, or Supplemental Security Income before this application

If you have applied for workers' compensation or public disability benefits

If you have served in the military, including the dates of service

If you ever earned Social Security credits while working in another country

Your marital status and spouse's name, date of birth, and Social Security number (for each marriage)

Date and location of each marriage and the disillusionment date

Your total earnings in all years since 1978

If you were employed or self-employed in the current and last year

The amount of earnings in the current and last year

If you will receive wages after the date you became unable to work

Besides filling out the application, you will need a copy of your Social Security card, your birth certificate (for proof of age), your checking and savings account information (for direct deposit of benefits), and your last W-2 form (Wage and Tax Statement). The application will ask for past employment information, your medical history, the names of all the medications you take, and the nature of your disability. Social Security will request copies of treatment records or the names of all the doctors who have been treating you. (It is helpful to your case if you have been treated by one main doctor, over a long period of time, who has been diligent about documenting your visits.)

Fast Fact _____

When applying for disability, you must be committed to being patient and to seeing the process through. Many people find that it is just too frustrating and difficult, and give up before their application makes it through the system. If you are truly disabled and unable to work, it is important that you move through the steps of application, taking it one day at a time.

Stages of Consideration

After you file your application for disability, your case is sent to a disability examiner at the Disability Determination agency in your state. This individual, working with a doctor, makes the initial decision on the claim within 90 to 120 days. If the claim is denied and you request reconsideration within 60 days, the case is then sent to another disability examiner at the Disability Determination agency. There, it goes through much the same process. Usually it takes up to four months to get a response at this stage of consideration.

If a claim is denied at reconsideration, you may then request a hearing. At this point, the case is sent to the office of Hearings and Appeals where it will eventually be referred to an administrative law judge who works for Social Security. It takes 6 months to 1½ years to see an administrative law judge. This judge will make an independent decision about the claim.

One of the biggest mistakes claimants make when trying to obtain disability benefits is failing to appeal, or if they do appeal, they fail to do it within the 60-day period. Additionally, many claimants fail to maintain a consistent treatment relationship with their health-care professionals. Medical treatment records provide the most important evidence of disability in a Social Security disability case.

The first step, however, is the process of filling out all the forms and collecting the necessary backup information. Scott Davis, Esq., a leading fibromyalgia Social Security attorney out of Phoenix, Arizona, recommends that you implement the following five tips:

Tip 1: Please do not write a book!

SSA does not give you a lot of room to answer the application questions, and that is good. Always answer the question honestly, but stick to the point.

Tip 2: Presume you are having a bad day when providing answers.

Remember, a critical issue in a Social Security disability case is always what activity level you are capable of *sustaining on a regular and continuing basis* (that is, a five-day workweek). The issue is never what you can do for only one day. Never forget: the issue is always what level of activity you can sustain on a daily basis, week after week.

Tip 3: Always focus on the "frequency, severity, and duration" of your symptoms and limitations.

Critical issues in your Social Security disability case are your symptoms and limitations (for example, pain, fatigue, concentration problems, or inability to maintain any activity for a reasonable period of time). You should mention all the diagnoses that have even a small impact on your inability to work, but you should use 5 percent of the allotted space to reference diagnoses and 95 percent to discuss how they limit not only your ability to work, but also your ability to function on a daily basis.

Tip 4: Completely resist the urge to be the perfectionist you are!

Before you became ill you may have been an organized perfectionist who was incredibly productive. Many people with fibromyalgia are unable to work due to concentration problems, memory impairment, and brain fog. The way you answer the application questions tells a lot about the severity of your concentration and memory problems.

Tip 5: If psychological issues play even a small part in preventing you from working, you must report them on the forms.

Although the primary reason you are unable to work may be due to a physical diagnosis, don't overlook the psychological issues that often arise after years of dealing with chronic pain and fatigue. Tell SSA if you believe that a psychological diagnosis plays a part in your inability to work. It is fine to state that it is "secondary to" or "as a result of" dealing with your chronic physical symptoms and limitations.

The Role of an Attorney

It is reasonable to consult with a disability attorney as soon as you decide to file a disability claim. Often, the information you provide the SSA without the assistance of a knowledgeable attorney will be used by the SSA or a judge at a later time to deny your claim. In many cases, the development of unfocused evidence can be avoided or mitigated if a knowledgeable disability attorney is involved from the beginning of your case. It is usually to your advantage to hire an attorney sooner than later.

A second part of your consideration should be that in most cases you only pay the attorney if and when your claim is approved. The SSA sets the attorney's fees, so you can be sure you are not overcharged for an attorney's services. Unfortunately, statistically your claim is very likely to be denied by SSA during the first two stages of review. If you have legal representation, you can develop a strategy to maximize your odds of winning. Overall, most good attorneys win between 75 and 90 percent of their cases.

What Is the Role of Your Health-Care Professional?

The key to a successful disability claim is the medical report. Joshua Potter, Esq., who practices law in Pasadena, California, points out, "It is critical to have the support of your treating health-care professional." So what happens to you if your health-care professional does not want to get involved or is not well educated in writing a disability report that satisfies the standards that SSA applies in evaluating medical evidence? This situation is serious and unfortunately not unusual, because SSA does not typically furnish health-care professionals with a full set of evaluation criteria. If a health-care professional is not well informed about the SSA's definition of disability, is not well versed as to how to meet the SSA's criteria for disability, or thinks that disability is always permanent, it is less likely that you will receive your health-care professional's support. You must overcome these obstacles.

Picture This/Lessons Learned

Picture This:

What strategies can your attorney help you with? Attorney Scott Davis provided an example to answer this question:

"Several weeks ago, SSA set up an appointment for one of my clients to see its doctor. My client's case was at the initial stage of review. I objected to the examination and would not let her go because her own doctor supported her claim. (I had personally spoken with him early in the case.) I arranged for her doctor to do the examination and as a result her claim was approved due to his opinions! I knew the doctor SSA chose and had rarely seen him conclude that someone was disabled. Sadly, had she not known any better and gone to the examination with SSA's doctor, her claim would certainly have been denied. However, her claim was approved because we had a strategy and implemented it!"

Lessons Learned:

Be sure that you are working with an attorney that is knowledgeable about SSDI, is experienced in representing people with fibromyalgia, and is willing to work with your health-care professional, if appropriate.

Initially, you will have to talk with your health-care professional about supporting your claim. It is important that your physician understands the definition of disability according to the SSA definition. (Often, health-care professionals are much stricter with their definition than is the SSA standard.) You will need to be cautious about the words you use to discuss your health situation. If you claim *permanent* disability, or state that you *are* disabled, it can hurt your relationship with your physician. It is his decision whether you are unable to do any kind of work. A good attorney will be able to communicate with your health-care professionals without including your emotional bias.

When you meet with your health-care professional, remember to keep it simple, and even though this can be a very emotional subject, try to stay calm and cooperative when discussing disability with your physician. It is essential that you have been seeing this physician long enough that he or she is well versed about your case. Be sure you express that you feel *currently* unable to sustain full-time work, but that you plan to go back to work as soon as it is possible. Most health-care professionals are willing to support temporary disability (18 to 24 months), as long as you are making an effort to improve your quality of health. You might even want to suggest that the two of you develop a plan that will help ensure improvement in your fibromyalgia over the next two years.

Although your health-care professional may see this process as a heavy reporting burden, with a properly designed chart this information can be obtained quickly. At a trial, the value of such an accurate and complete record is immeasurable. Joshua Potter explains that every patient visit should result in entries concerning physical capabilities for lifting, bending, and carrying (verified with measured weight); time durations for sitting, standing, and walking (by history); psychosocial and adaptive behavior, including the ability to interact appropriately with others, follow instructions, and adhere to a regular schedule; and the complexity of depressive symptoms. Not only are height, weight, and blood pressure essential elements in charting, but so are adaptive reactions, physical capabilities, and functional deficits.

Attorney Joshua Potter also advises that the health-care professional's narrative report include the following:

> History—A description of the patient's work history, demonstrating familiarity with past work. It should include the work's physical and intellectual demands.

> Examination—Reference to the patient's medical chart, including a report on pain and the side effects of pain medication; an assessment of mental health; a report on measured physical capacity; and physical findings, including a reference to tolerance for sitting, walking, and lifting.

> Discussion—A review of objective physical test results and clinical observations; a discussion of pain, specifying the activities that exacerbate the pain; support for the prognosis, accompanied by an indication that the health-care professional has seen many similar cases and is familiar with the pathology of the disease; the health-care professional's allegations as to his expertise in this field, and that the patient is not malingering or seeking secondary gain; as well as a statement strongly confirming the diagnosis and stating that the symptoms are consistent with diagnosis.

How to Win Your Case

You can do many things to help ensure that you win your disability case. To get through the process, be sure that you have the involvement of a well-informed, supportive health-care professional, a knowledgeable attorney, and family members who are willing to assist you and to see that you are mentally prepared to be persistent throughout the entire process. You do not win your case proving that you have fibromyalgia, but rather that you are physically incapable of performing your past job functions and all other types of work. (Note: these rules vary for persons over the age of 50.) Your case must focus on proving that there is a presence of a medically determinable condition that prevents you from substantial gainful employment. In cases concerning fibromyalgia, one of the more vital points that you need to prove is that your illness prevents you from *regular* work attendance.

You may not have to complete all the steps in the disability application process if your claim is approved at one of the earlier stages; outlined below, however, here is the complete succession of steps.

Fast Fact _____

Seventy-five percent of all disability applicants will initially be denied benefits! Half of those denied will give up and not appeal the denial. However, 53 percent of the applicants who persevere to a hearing before an administrative law judge will obtain benefits!

Disability Steps*

Process	Participant
File initial application	Filled out and completed by claimant.
Response to application	Letter sent to claimant from SSA (application approved or denied).
Request for reconsideration	Filed by claimant within 60 days of rejection (must be within 60 days!).
Claimant's medical chart	Health-care professional supplies claimant's chart if copied and forwarded to SSA requested by SSA.
Physical examination	Performed by SSA physician. (Your attorney might be able to have this examination performed by your own health-care professional.)

continues

Disability Steps*   (continued)

Process	Participant
Response to reconsideration	SSA provides its decision on the reconsideration request.
Request for hearing	Claimant requests a hearing for reconsideration within 60 days.
Updated medical chart	Supplied by physician. Be prepared to forward it to SSA.
Trial	Claimant, attorney, and physician participate before an administrative law judge.
Judge's decision	Attorney files an appeal to the Appeals Court within 60 days.
Lawsuit	Filed by the attorney with the United States District Court within 60 days. (Attorney must have license to practice in District Court.)

Joshua Potter, Esq., fmscommunity.org/potter.htm

Attorney Scott Davis points out that for your claim to be approved, "… 5 percent of your time is spent on discussing the diagnosis and 95 percent is spent determining the frequency, severity, and duration of symptoms and limitations, and whether they prevent you from performing all work." It's very important to not get too caught up in the diagnosis part of the case, but to concentrate on the limitations that keep you from being able to work. Often a person with fibromyalgia also suffers from other illnesses, such as migraine headaches, depression, or quantifiable sleep disorders. Do not forget to include these illnesses and their limitations in your medical chart and application narrative.

So how do you document these limitations? To begin, you must accurately express to your health-care professional your symptoms and what they limit you from doing. For example, "I am experiencing extreme daily fatigue, so if I get up for more than one hour at a time, I become incapacitated by the resulting pain, cognitive dysfunction, and physical weakness, which causes me to go back to bed for the rest of the day. I experience this level of fatigue at least four days out of the week."

Make sure that your health-care professional notes your statements in your medical record. If you are not sure whether specific information is being logged in your chart, you are entitled to request a copy of your chart from the physician's office. If you notice that important information is missing, you may want to tactfully approach your health-care professional and explain the importance of documenting your case.

It is easy to be short of patience when you are in pain. However, people talk, and what they say can influence what is written in your medical chart. Remember to be nice to everyone in the doctor's office, even the appointment secretary. Most nurses and doctors have a very limited amount of time to write in your chart. For this reason it is not surprising to learn that most health-care professionals rarely write more than five sentences about your health complaints. Choose your words carefully, and speak no faster than the nurse or doctor can write. If it is not written down, it will not be considered in court.

Fast Fact

In most cases, people with fibromyalgia are real "go-getters" before the illness sets in. Even after being limited by their symptoms, many people with fibromyalgia tend to overexert themselves. When you start stressing about the disability case, it is important to focus on protecting your health and save your limited energy for issues related to the case. Often people going through the disability process find their symptoms getting worse because of the stressful process.

Next, you will want to create a journal to keep track of your symptoms and limitations. You can make copies of these notes to take with you when you go see your health-care professional. Do not give these pages to your doctor, because if your chart looks like a journal, it will have less credibility as a medical chart. Use your journal to refresh your memory before you see the doctor. This will help you to remember what has been going on over a long period of time, and it will save time when you are at your doctor's office.

And the final most important element to winning your case is to never give up. If you get discouraged and quit, then you have no way of winning your case. As Scott Davis, Esq., points out, "The only way you can win is if you keep appealing to the next level in the SSA process."

Disability Questions and Answers

The following questions regarding SSDI were presented to and answered by Scott Davis, attorney at law.

Are other members of my family qualified for benefits on my claim?

Your spouse, who is age 62 or older, or any age if he or she is caring for a child of yours who is under the age of 16 or disabled, will also qualify for benefits.

Your disabled widow or widower aged 50 or older. The disability must have started before your death or within seven years after your death. (If your widow or widower caring for your children receives Social Security checks, she or he is eligible if she or he becomes disabled before those payments end or within seven years after they end.)

Your unmarried son or daughter, including an adopted child, or, in some cases, a stepchild or grandchild. The child must be under age 18 or under age 19 if in high school full-time.

Your unmarried son or daughter, age 18 or older, if he or she has a disability that started before age 22.

Am I eligible for Medicare if I am approved for SSDI?

Yes. You will be eligible for Medicare 24 months after you have been receiving SSDI benefits. Medicare is a real bargain; the monthly premium is only $45.50.

If I have been self-employed, can I get SSDI if I become disabled?

Self-employed people who become disabled can receive SSDI if they have paid the federal government a sufficient amount of self-employment tax or FICA tax to qualify for SSDI coverage.

I am disabled, but I have plenty of money in the bank. Do I have to wait until this money is gone before I apply for Social Security disability benefits?

No. If you have worked in recent years or if you are applying for disabled widow's or widower's benefits or disabled adult child benefits, it does not matter how much money you have in the bank. There is no reason to wait to file the claim.

Do I have to be permanently disabled to get Social Security disability benefits?

No. You have to be disabled for at least a year or be expected to be disabled for at least a year.

How do I find an attorney to represent me on my Social Security disability claim?

The National Organization of Social Security Claimants' Representatives (NOSSCR) offers a referral service. You may call NOSSCR at 1-800-431-2804 during regular Eastern Time business hours. It can also be helpful to contact a fibromyalgia support group or national organization.

How far back will they pay benefits if I am found disabled?

For disability insurance benefits and for disabled widow's and widower's benefits, the benefits cannot begin until five months have passed after the person becomes disabled. In addition, benefits cannot be paid more than one year prior to the date of the claim.

What is the Social Security hearing like?

The hearings are fairly informal. The only people likely to be there are the judge, a secretary operating a tape recorder, the claimant, the claimant's attorney, and anyone else the claimant has brought with him or her. In some cases, the administrative law judge has a medical doctor or vocational expert present to testify at the hearing. There is no jury nor are there any spectators at the hearing.

If I get on Social Security disability benefits and get to feeling better and want to return to work, can I return to work?

Certainly you can return to work. Social Security wants individuals drawing disability benefits to return to work and gives them every encouragement to do so. For persons receiving disability insurance benefits, disabled widow's and widower's benefits, and disabled adult child benefits, full benefits may continue for a year after an individual returns to work. Even thereafter, an individual who has to stop work in the following three years can get back on Social Security disability benefits immediately without having to file a new claim.

I am already on Social Security disability benefits, but I am worried that my benefits will be stopped in the future. What are the chances of this happening?

Social Security is not supposed to cut off disability benefits for an individual unless his or her medical condition has improved. When Social Security reviews a case of someone already on Social Security disability benefits, it continues benefits in the vast majority of cases. In recent years, Social Security has been doing few reviews to determine whether individuals already on Social Security disability benefits are still disabled. This is changing and Social Security should be doing far more reviews in the next few years. However, the vast majority of individuals who are reviewed will see their Social Security disability benefits continued.

How Do I Get Back to Work?

Most individuals prefer to go back to work rather than try to live on disability benefits. To do this you need to be aware of the rules of the "work incentives" and "employment support" programs that provide cash benefits and Medicare while you attempt to work. Working on a trial basis is only available if you are receiving SSDI. The SSA's intention in creating the trial work period is to give you an opportunity to see whether you can go back to work without compromising your approved disability benefits. Everyone on SSDI is eligible to participate in the trial work period. The trial work period cannot begin before the month in which you file your application for disability benefits. You can participate in this program until you have accumulated 9 months of work within a 60-month period of time. This allows you to return to work and not be penalized by SSA. The SSA, however, may find that your disability has ended at any time during the trial work period if medical or other evidence shows that you are not disabled.

For more information, you can call toll-free 1-800-772-1213 and ask for the fact sheet "Ticket to Work and Work Incentives Improvement Act of 1999" (Publication No. 05-10060). The fact sheet also is available at www.socialsecurity.gov/work. For more information about Social Security work incentives, ask for a copy of the booklet "Working While Disabled...How We Can Help" (Publication No. 05-10095).

The Least You Need to Know

- ◆ The Social Security Administration has determined that fibromyalgia "can constitute medically determinable impairments within the meaning of the statute."

- ◆ Several kinds of disability programs exist, including state worker's compensation, private pension disability, public pension plans, and Social Security Disability Insurance (SSDI).

- ◆ To qualify for Social Security Disability Insurance, you have to meet Social Security's qualifications.

- ◆ As soon as you know that you are not capable of working any time in the next 12 months and that you have a valid disability case, you should contact the Social Security Administration (the SSA nationwide number is 1-800-772-1213) and request an application to apply for disability.

- ◆ When applying for disability, you must be committed to being patient and to seeing the process through.

- ◆ You can do many things to help ensure that you win your disability case. To get through the process, make sure that you have the involvement of a well-informed, supportive health-care professional, a knowledgeable attorney, and family members who are willing to suport you throughout the entire process.

Hope on the Horizon

In This Chapter

- ◆ Learning about new treatments and ones that might be approved in the near future
- ◆ Finding what new discoveries will mean to people with fibromyalgia
- ◆ Knowing the people who are working to help provide new options

Every day that you have to experience pain is one day too many. However, fibromyalgia is a complicated disorder and it will take extensive research to solve the mysteries behind its causes. The good news is that scientific interest in the field of disordered sensory processing is growing rapidly. Since the approval of Lyrica by the FDA, the pharmaceutical industry has become more interested in advancing fibromyalgia research and investigating better treatments for this disease. The extensive need for the development of new treatment options depends on carrying out more clinical trials, which will result in more drugs specifically approved to treat fibromyalgia. Even private research funding is growing, and with the new focus on physiological abnormalities in people with fibromyalgia, the next advances in research will help us to understand the underlying scientific basis for our symptoms including pain amplification.

When the pain is difficult to deal with, remember that in just the last couple of years our knowledge and the scientific interest in the understanding of fibromyalgia has increased faster than at any other time in history. In 1992, there were approximately 250 published scientific papers on fibromyalgia research; today there are more than 4,500. The process will continue to improve and the future will provide more answers.

What Promise Does the Future Hold?

As you discovered in this book, there are things you can do to help reduce fibromyalgia symptoms and improve overall quality of life. Over the past 20 years, the medical community has made incredible advances in its understanding and acceptance of fibromyalgia. You must always remember that the status of your illness will not remain stagnant. New options will be discovered, and you are not alone in your attempts to find relief. With millions of people dealing with this illness, others recognize the benefits of helping you return to a healthy, productive life. Experts agree that significant, unmet needs exist and that we must expand our knowledge of virtually every stage of fibromyalgia research and management.

Until recently, people with fibromyalgia have had to utilize off-label medications (drugs approved for other uses), but *specific medications* are now being approved as therapies for fibromyalgia. With the U.S. Food and Drug Administration in the process of approving multiple medications, as well as the development of more targeted therapies and their successes during clinical trials, specific treatment protocols are beginning to emerge. It is because researchers have made great strides in learning more about the causes of fibromyalgia that pharmaceutical manufacturers are pushing to develop products to address the basic components of the underlying symptoms.

Fast Fact _____

In the last couple of years, two major steps forward have happened: fibromyalgia researchers now have a better understanding of what might contribute to the cause of fibromyalgia (that is, disordered sensory processing at a central level), and they are starting to refer to it as a disease rather than an illness. The new medications approved by the FDA are still for symptom management. As research moves forward and we better understand the underlying mechanisms that cause the symptoms of fibromyalgia, scientists will develop treatment options that will help "cure" the physiological abnormalities, rather than just treat the symptoms. The fact that investigators now refer to fibromyalgia as a disease gives further legitimacy to these symptoms and will increase research interest in this "invisible" disease.

Leslie Crofford, M.D., now at the University of Kentucky, and her colleagues from the University of Michigan have presented research outcome data on pregabalin (Lyrica) as an effective and safe treatment for pain in people with fibromyalgia. A third pharmacological agent, duloxetine (Cymbalta), studied by Leslie Arnold, M.D., in conjunction with the Duloxetine Fibromyalgia Trial Group, has been approved for the treatment of depression. It, however, has proved to be an effective and safe treatment for fibromyalgia in patients with or without depression. Studies have shown that duloxetine has a direct effect on pain and is now used in the treatment of diabetic neuropathy. Now with two FDA-approved products for treating fibromyalgia, the hope of these new drugs is that we are entering into a time when scientific research will offer more options as therapies to help millions of people with fibromyalgia.

Pregabalin (Lyrica)

Pregabalin received FDA approval for the treatment of fibromyalgia on June 21, 2007. It was previously approved in the United Sates for the treatment of neuropathic pain associated with diabetic peripheral neuropathy, generalized anxiety disorder, and as an adjunctive therapy for partial seizures in patients with epilepsy. In scientific studies, pregabalin demonstrated improvement in pain in patients with fibromyalgia. Data also suggested that it can help improve sleep and fatigue levels.

Developer: Pfizer, Inc.

Stage of research: Besides FDA approval in the United States, Pfizer reported that the European Commission granted approval of pregabalin (Lyrica) in all EU member states for the treatment of peripheral neuropathic pain and as an adjunctive therapy for partial seizures in patients with epilepsy.

About the drug: Pregabalin is derived from Neurontin (gabapentin), a second-generation anticonvulsant medication, approved in 1993 for the treatment of epileptic seizures. Anticonvulsants are believed to work in part by enhancing the actions of a brain chemical called GABA (gamma-aminobutyric acid). GABA is a neurotransmitter, a chemical that transmits messages between the nerve cells of the brain. GABA inhibits the transmission of nerve signals, thereby reducing nervous excitation and pain.

Expected outcome: Recent studies prove that pregabalin is effective and safe for patients to use up to 450 milligrams a day for reducing pain (pain was reduced by 50 percent from the baseline in approximately 30 percent of the fibromyalgia research participants) and for helping with associated symptoms (including sleep and fatigue) in patients with fibromyalgia.

def•i•ni•tion

The term **mean pain score** is the level of pain that the patient reports. If a treatment is successful, then a patient will have an improvement in their mean pain score.

Drug efficacy: Pregabalin had previously been shown to be effective in trials for neuropathic pain and generalized anxiety. Fibromyalgia patients treated with pregabalin showed significant improvement in their *mean pain score* and their sleep index score. About one third of the fibromyalgia patients had 50 percent or greater pain relief. It was effective in reducing pain within one week. The majority of patients noted positive improvement in their sleep, fatigue, and general health.

Duloxetine (Cymbalta)

Duloxetine (Cymbalta) After successfully completing Phase III of clinical trials, a New Drug Application (NDA) was filed with the U.S. Food and Drug Administration for the approval of duloxetine in the treatment of fibromyalgia. It received approval in June of 2008. It was previously approved in the United States in August 2004 for the treatment of major depressive disorder and later for treatment of diabetic neuropathy.

Developer: Eli Lilly and Company

Stage of research: The results of clinical trials conducted at 18 centers, including the University of Cincinnati College of Medicine, Indiana University Medical School, and Harvard Medical School, to evaluate the use of duloxetine to treat pain and tiredness in patients with fibromyalgia were positive. The results showed significant improvement in pain and tiredness, independent of the drug's effect on mood.

About the drug: Duloxetine (Cymbalta) is part of a new class of medications known as Norepinephrine Serotonin Reuptake Inhibitors, or NSRIs. It is considered an antidepressant dual noradrenalin and 5HT reuptake inhibitor, and it works by inhibiting the reuptake of both serotonin and norepinephrine. It is also FDA approved for the treatment of diabetic neuropathy, an extremely painful condition.

Expected outcome: Multiple study outcome data revealed that duloxetine is an effective treatment in reducing fibromyalgia symptomology. It was beneficial in lowering pain scores as well as tiredness, and it helped with sleep. It also reduced the number of tender points in fibromyalgia volunteers taking part in the scientific studies.

Drug efficacy: According to Lesley M. Arnold, M.D., who coordinated the clinical trials, when evaluating pervasive pain to tiredness to tenderness, the female fibromyalgia patients treated with duloxetine improved significantly over those treated with a placebo. One of the most dramatic changes was in the reduction of the number of tender points (i.e., places on the body where it hurts to touch and that are used to diagnosis fibromyalgia).

Milnacipran

This drug has been commercially available for six years in Japan and parts of Europe, South America, and Asia for treating depression.

Developer: Cypress Bioscience, Inc., and Forest Laboratories, Inc.

Stage of research: After successfully completing Phase III of clinical trials, a New Drug Application (NDA) was filed with the U.S. Food and Drug Administration for the approval of Milnacipran in the treatment of fibromyalgia in December of 2007. It is hoped that it will be approved sometime during 2008.

Dr. Daniel Clauw, director, Chronic Pain and Fatigue Research Center at the University of Michigan, has been involved in the research of Milnacipran, which has shown major improvements in fibromyalgia symptoms. "It is impressive to see such a significant improvement … in this patient population," commented Dr. Clauw. Milnacipran is expected to be approved by the FDA in late 2008.

About the drug: According to Jay D. Kranzler, M.D., Ph.D., chairman of the board and chief executive officer of Cypress, "Milnacipran is a novel compound that exerts its effect by inhibiting the reuptake of both norepinephrine and serotonin, two neurotransmitters known to play an essential role in regulating pain and mood. With its unique pharmacology, the compound has the potential to provide relief of multiple fibromyalgia symptoms by acting on more than one neuropathway. Furthermore, the fact that Milnacipran has little activity on other receptor systems means it results in a favorable side-effect profile."

Expected outcome: To receive FDA approval to make Milnacipran available to the fibromyalgia community.

Drug efficacy: Milnacipran reduced pain by 50 percent or more in about one third of the patients involved in clinical trials. The majority of patients reported an overall clinical improvement in their fibromyalgia. Milnacipran has also been shown to reduce fatigue in fibromyalgia patients, as well as improve depressed moods.

According to Stuart Silverman, M.D., Cedars-Sinai Medical Center, and clinical professor of medicine and rheumatology at David Geffen School of Medicine UCLA, "The exciting news for people with fibromyalgia is that there are many new therapies which show promise in randomized, controlled clinical trials. There is an early suggestion that some of these therapies not only reduce pain, but also treat the syndrome. Others are effective for a particular symptom of fibromyalgia such as sleep. It is likely we may combine multiple therapies in the future to target multiple points in the pain pathways. The best results are likely to require pharmacologic and nonpharmacologic treatments."

Research Directions

Dr. I. Jon Russell, M.D., at the University of Texas Health Science Center in San Antonio, has been involved in answering some of the broad questions that will help us understand the possible causes of fibromyalgia. For example, he and other researchers have found that people with fibromyalgia have elevated levels of substance P (a pain neurotransmitter) found in the spinal cord. To expand upon this finding, Dr. Russell is researching the benefits of normalizing the level of substance P with certain drugs. The answers to these types of far-reaching questions could have critical importance on the future management of fibromyalgia. With new discoveries, there will be ways to treat and prevent the chronic amount of discomfort people with this condition experience.

Fast Fact

Although only three drugs are mentioned here, many pharmacy companies are currently researching multiple-perspective pharmacological treatments for fibromyalgia. Others include dopamine agonists currently used in the treatment of Parkinson's disease and restless legs syndrome, as well as sodium oxybate, a sleep medication.

New discoveries will provide fibromyalgia sufferers with many benefits, including the following:

◆ Health-care professionals now have additional therapeutic options to recommend to their patients.

◆ Pharmaceutical marketing programs are raising awareness about fibromyalgia and helping inform physicians about the condition.

◆ The FDA approval of a drug with an indication for fibromyalgia is helping promote the legitimacy of fibromyalgia as a disease and diagnosis.

◆ Researchers are beginning to have a new understanding of the mechanisms of pain.

In developing specialized drugs to treat fibromyalgia, the goal is still to find products that have limited or no side effects and work on multiple symptoms. Because fibromyalgia is now recognized as the second most commonly diagnosed condition by rheumatologists in the United States, the medical community must find ways to appropriately and efficiently serve the needs of their fibromyalgia patients.

The American College of Rheumatology is interested in encouraging new medical students to consider a specialty in rheumatology, and pharmaceutical companies are exploring their options for finding fibromyalgia treatments. Part of the research includes evaluating existing drugs such as Provigil (which may reduce fatigue associated with fibromyalgia and chronic fatigue syndrome) and Mirapex (which helps people with fibromyalgia produce more dopamine, eliminating spasms related to restless legs syndrome, and provides major improvement in other fibromyalgia symptoms). Both have been approved for other uses and are being studied for effectiveness in treating fibromyalgia symptoms.

Another exciting development in the understanding and future of fibromyalgia is the recent development of the Fibromyalgia Epidemiological Task Force. Chaired by Robert Bennett, M.D., with members representing an elite group of fibromyalgia researchers, the Task Force implemented a multi-center survey to collect statistical data that will help guide future research and give us a better understanding of the patient's perspective, beliefs, and expectations. This far-reaching questionnaire delved into areas such as gender disparity, age at onset, symptom fluctuation, symptom relief, emotional coping, financial burden, support systems, relationship impact, and so on. The data has been collected and analyzed and the Task Force is implementing longitudinal interventional studies to create a "National Fibromyalgia Blueprint" that will chart a plan for future research and patient assistance. On March 9, 2007, the first paper, "An Internet survey of 2,596 people with fibromyalgia" was published in the BMC Musculoskeletal Disorders located on the BioMed website, regarding the data from this study. Several more articles are being created from the information collected in this survey for future publications. Based on the responses collected in the first study, an "Epi II" investigation is being developed that will fulfill and clarify some of the findings from the first research project.

Other interesting fibromyalgia studies include …

- ◆ **Functional MRI (fMRI).** Dr. Dan Clauw's group at the University of Michigan is continuing fMRI studies, comparing responses of fibromyalgia patients to a pain stimulus to healthy control subjects. In the MRI equipment study, volunteers are subjected to pressure placed on the thumbnail. To fibromyalgia subjects, this pressure is perceived as a painful stimulus. The same pressure is applied to the healthy control volunteers without a painful response. The MRI pictures show that the fibromyalgia patients have areas in the brain that light up in response to the thumb pressure, indicating a painful response, whereas the healthy controls do not show this activity in the brain. The significance of these studies is the demonstration of how people with fibromyalgia perceive pain compared to healthy people and for the first time scientists actually have pictures showing this comparison. The fMRIs are providing researchers with information about abnormal pain processing in the brain that has been theorized to be a major cause of discomfort in fibromyalgia patients.

♦ **PET Scans.** A 2008 paper by Dr. Patrick Wood describes his imaging work at McGill University in Montreal, Canada, the world's epicenter in pain imaging. This study was undertaken to check out his theory regarding diminished dopamine (a neurotransmitter that is involved in Parkinson's disease) in fibromyalgia patients. PET scans revealed that a painful stimulus in fibromyalgia patients was recorded in the brain much differently than healthy controls. He also was able to demonstrate changes in the brain in fibromyalgia subjects compared to controls. Imaging is finally giving pictures of changes in the brains of fibromyalgia patients that, for years, have been theoretically conceived. This new kind of science should help researchers develop better treatment programs that will help with fibromyalgia symptoms.

♦ **Patient-Reported Outcomes Measurement Information System (PROMIS).** This is a National Institutes of Health study that is being conducted at the University of Michigan with collaboration of offsite locations, including the National Fibromyalgia Association, helping to collect data. It is hoped that the results of this scientific investigation will help doctors understand how fibromyalgia affects patients and how better treatment protocols might be developed based on their responses to hundreds of questions. It will take approximately three years to complete, but the benefits to fibromyalgia patients should be outstanding.

♦ **Overlapping Conditions.** As all patients who have fibromyalgia already know, several other illnesses are usually present as well. Irritable bowel syndrome (IBS), restless legs syndrome, Sjögren's syndrome (dry mouth and eyes), chronic fatigue, headaches, cognition problems (fibro fog), TMJ, interstitial cystitis (IC, a bladder condition), sleep problems including apnea, and myofascial pain syndrome are just some of the added conditions that fibromyalgia patients endure. Many of these illnesses have the same mechanisms that cause pain and other symptoms. Scientists are working on studies looking at similarities in these diseases with the hope that a better understanding of how these overlapping conditions are related could help them develop new and better treatment modalities.

A Future of Hope and Understanding

Always remember that you can and will have improvement in your fibromyalgia symptoms by implementing your own personalized self-management plan. If you ever want a reminder, you can read and reread the following expressions of hope by people who care and understand.

Words of encouragement:

"Although fibromyalgia may change your life, it can be a change for the better. When you were healthy, you probably got involved in many activities ... some because they interested you and some because you felt obligated. Now you must choose your activities carefully and use your limited energy to focus on those things that are most important to you. Many things in life may catch your eye or spark your interest, but very few will touch your heart. Pursue what touches your heart."

—Karen Lee Richards, cofounder, National Fibromyalgia Association

"When I first became ill, I used to rant, 'I want my life back!' I felt as though the rug had been pulled out from under me. I had a happy life of a single, busy emergency-room nurse and mom of three teenaged sons—I was in two car accidents in 1987 and diagnosed with fibromyalgia after the second one. I lost my freedom, my home, my income, and my self-confidence. Fortunately, I met some of my closest friends because of fibromyalgia, and by serving on the NFA board of directors, together we have built a source of hope and self-realization. Now I rant, 'I want my life forward,' because I can't wait to see what is around the next corner!"

—Sharon Squires, R.N.

"Hope and understanding are synonymous with one another—with an understanding of this disorder you will find more hope. Continuing to learn all you can about fibromyalgia will help the light at the end of the tunnel become bigger and brighter."

—Errol T. Landy, FM Supporter

"Dealing with fibromyalgia syndrome has been a complicated process for twentieth-century medicine because of widely conflicting opinions about this condition. The reasons for the postured stereotypes are buried deep in the fabric of belief system anchoring. An optimistic confidence in a more insightful future is based on the application of scientific methodologies to the questions at hand."

—I. Jon Russell, M.D., Ph.D., associate professor of medicine, director, University Clinical Research Center, University of Texas Health Science Center

"Just when I think that I'm at the bottom and can't take the pain anymore, I remember hearing that weak voice on the phone saying 'Thank you for saving my life,' and I just melt. In 2000 when the National Fibromyalgia Association (NFA) assisted *Dateline NBC* and Maria Shriver to present a segment on the dilemma of fibromyalgia to millions of viewers across the TV waves … the phone lines at NFA lit up. But that one phone call that I answered was a lady whose family had completely abandoned her. Her children had been taken away from her, and she was ready to give up, but she then saw the *Dateline* story. It was because of the show that the woman's family called her to say they had seen the show and finally understood why she was so sick. Her mother, who had not spoken to her in 15 years, called and said she was coming over to help her and bring her children over. The story had a happy ending. It meant so much to me to know that I was in the right place, doing the right thing, and that even though I have fibromyalgia, I can help others and help spread awareness.

—Karin Amour, NFA, Board of Directors

"A depressed spirit saps one's strength, but a happy mind is good medicine."

—Proverbs 17:22

"Health can be influenced by developing lifestyle qualities that are balanced and positive. Be persistent, while practicing patience. Learn when to push yourself to accomplish something, and when to rest to protect your health. Focus on a brighter future, but do not let your expectations turn into disappointments. Be kind to yourself, and focus on your faith. Happiness will be attainable."

—Marina Chandler, Fibromyalgia Support Leader

"Fibromyalgia is a problem of hypersensitivity, so the treatment goal is hardiness. Each person with fibromyalgia should work toward their own personal best. It is important that you believe that improvement can happen."

—Stuart L. Silverman, M.D., F.A.C.P., F.A.C.R.

"There was a time when I couldn't get out of bed. My hopes and dreams were put on hold and I wondered if I would ever be able to participate in the activities of life again. I was frozen by pain and fear and I just laid there waiting for things to change. Then one day I remembered an experience I had when I was living in England. I was with a group of people who asked me if I would like to go out for a walk. As I peered out through the window of the building I noticed sheets of rain hitting the panes of glass. Go for a walk, were they crazy? I immediately protested, wondering how they hadn't realized that it was pouring rain outside. My new English friends just laughed. 'If you wait for it to stop raining in England, you will never go outside!' In this memory, I realized that if I waited for the pain to go away, I would never get my life back. Today, I pursue my dreams and follow my hopes. There are days when it is raining and days when it is sunny and beautiful, but no matter what "kind" of day it is, I love taking a walk!"

—Lynne Matallana, President and Cofounder, National Fibromyalgia Association

Take the time to write down your own words of inspiration. You can also have your family, friends, and health-care professionals add to this list of thoughts with their own words of encouragement and positive inspiration.

My Final Words to You

Time has a wonderful way of healing. Not just because your body can heal with the passage of time, but emotionally you can learn how to focus more and more on the positive. Memories from the past change and happy memories rise up above the more negative ones, forcing the difficult times out from the forefront of our attention. Although I will never completely forget the misery and enormous challenges of the years 1995–1997—when fibromyalgia forced me to bed, I was unable to participate in life, and getting through each day of pain had to be taken one minute at a time— today those memories don't incapacitate me with fear, but rather provide me with the strength and inspiration to move forward with a new way of life, always recognizing how wonderful it is that life is constantly offering us new opportunities.

No longer are we faced with a medical community that rejects our pain and suffering; in most cases, there are health-care professionals in your community ready and able to help you find ways to improve your symptoms. And there are individuals, corporations, and organizations that are putting the understanding and treatment of fibromyalgia as their top priority. Now that the wheels of motion have been put in place, there is no turning back. Ignorance will be overshadowed by research, and human suffering will no longer be hidden away because of feelings of guilt and embarrassment.

When I finally did get out of bed and started finding ways to help me to once again become a functioning and contributing member of society, I had no idea what my future was going to hold. I didn't know what to expect and I certainly didn't know what to dream for. But today I can tell you with complete confidence that you should not be afraid of the future. You should dream, even those that seem to be the most impossible of dreams. Change may come slowly, but with the power of perseverance, you can truly amaze even yourself.

The Least You Need to Know

- Experts agree that significant unmet needs exist and that we must expand our knowledge of virtually every stage of fibromyalgia research and management.

- With the development of more targeted therapies, and their successes during clinical trials, specific therapies for fibromyalgia will soon be available.

- Fibromyalgia symptoms do improve when you implement a self-management plan.

- Understanding and treating fibromyalgia is a priority for numerous individuals, organizations, and corporations.

- It is important that you believe improvement can happen.

Glossary

acetaminophen   A type of pain reliever that does not contain aspirin and does not need a prescription.

allodynia   When something, such as a light touch on your skin, causes pain when it shouldn't.

American College of Rheumatology (ACR)   The official organization for health-care professionals who treat arthritis and other rheumatic diseases. This organization established the criteria for diagnosing fibromyalgia.

analgesic   A drug that helps reduce or eliminate the perception of pain.

antidepressant   A prescription medication that is prescribed to relieve moodiness and depression. Some antidepressants can also promote sleep and help relieve pain.

arthritis   Joint pain. A diagnosis of arthritis means that you are experiencing joint inflammation that causes pain, swelling, stiffness, and redness in any joint in the body. Note: Unlike arthritis, fibromyalgia is not an inflammatory illness, nor does it cause degeneration of joint or connective tissues (for example, cartilage).

central nervous system   Nerve tissue that is located in the brain and the spinal cord.

chronic disease An illness characterized by alterations in normal functioning that cannot be reversed by medical treatment. However, most chronic illnesses can be effectively managed using medical treatment and patient education. Education for the cause of your illnesses and for the changes in your behavior (for example, coping skills) may reduce symptoms and can help produce a better quality of life.

circadian rhythm The daily rhythm that your body adjusts to in order to carry out essential biological functions.

cognition Information processing by the brain/mind; examples include learning/memory, concentration, and executive function (i.e., decision making).

comorbidity The presence of one or more disorders (or diseases) in addition to a primary disease or disorder. Examples of common comorbid conditions in fibromyalgia include restless legs syndrome, irritable bowel syndrome, migraine headaches, and interstitial cystitis.

connective tissue The tissue that binds together and supports the various structures of the body.

cytokines Chemical messengers of the immune system.

diagnostic criteria A predetermined set of symptoms or physical findings identified by a physical examination or laboratory tests. They are used to accurately identify specific illnesses consistently by health-care providers.

disease A condition that affects an organism and impairs its normal physiological functioning. Sometimes this term is only used for conditions where there is structural or functional change in the organs or tissues involved.

disorder Some form of abnormal health.

dopamine A neurotransmitter that reacts similarly to adrenaline. It affects the part of the brain that controls movement and the ability to experience pleasure and pain.

enzyme A protein that accelerates chemical reactions.

FDA United States Food and Drug Administration (FDA); the federal agency responsible for protecting the public health by assuring the safety, efficacy, and security of human and veterinary drugs, biological products, medical devices, the country's food supply, cosmetics, and products that emit radiation. The FDA is also responsible for advancing the public health by helping to speed innovations that make medicines and foods more effective, safer, and more affordable; and helping the public get the accurate, science-based information they need to use medicines and foods to improve their health.

fibro fog (cognitive dysfunction)   A term that is popular among people with fibromyalgia that refers to a cluster of cognitive symptoms that may hinder an individual's ability to function effectively. These symptoms include memory loss, difficulty in concentrating, confusion, and disorientation.

flare   A period of time (with a start and a finish) when symptoms reoccur, becoming worse and then slowly starting to improve again. A flare does not mean that your fibromyalgia is getting worse.

functional neuroimaging   The use of neuroimaging technology to measure aspects of brain function, often with a view to understanding the relationship between the activity in certain brain areas and aspects of human experience such as information processing (cognition), motor function (control of movement), or pain perception. Most medical imaging is used to evaluate anatomical structures (e.g., x-rays or CT scans for bones; MRI for soft tissues, including the brain); functional neuroimaging allows observations about the activity (function) of the brain. A variety of technologies are used in neuroimaging depending on the type of function that researchers want to evaluate. These include functional magnetic resonance imaging (fMRI), positron emission tomography (PET), and magnetoencephalography (MEG).

genetic predisposition   The genetic susceptibility to inherit a specific characteristic or disease.

hormones   Chemical messengers that include insulin, estrogen, thyroid, steroids, progesterone, and testosterone.

immune system   The body's system that defends against foreign substances.

interstitial cystitis   A medical condition characterized by chronic or recurring discomfort or pain in the bladder. Symptoms may include mild discomfort, pressure, tenderness, or intense pain in the bladder and surrounding pelvic area. Other symptoms include an urgent need to urinate, a frequent need to urinate, or a combination of these symptoms.

metabolism   The body's ongoing physical and chemical processes, which build up body tissue while eating food, and break down while expending energy.

myalgia   Pain that occurs in the muscles.

myofascial pain syndrome   Pain similar to fibromyalgia pain, but located in only one area or region of the body.

neuralgia   A painful condition caused by disorders of the nervous system.

neurally mediated hypotension   Abnormally low blood pressure (hypotension) related to an abnormal reflex interaction between the brain and cardiovascular system (i.e., heart and blood vessels). The brain normally responds to cues from the body to determine blood pressure. Neurally mediated hypotension occurs when the nerves controlling blood pressure fail to respond appropriately. Also known as the fainting reflex, neurocardiogenic syncope, vasodepressor syncope, the vaso-vagal reflex, and autonomic dysfunction.

neuroendocrine dysfunction   A dysfunction of the endocrine (hormonal) system(s) related to changes in the function of brain structures that control hormone release (e.g., the hypothalamus). The endocrine system is a collection of hormone-releasing glands that are controlled by a "master gland" called the *pituitary gland*. The pituitary gland is, in turn, controlled by a brain center called the *hypothalamus*.

neuroendocrine system   A complex system of brain structures and glands that help regulate the release of a large number of hormones, steroids, and neuropeptides that contribute to the transmission and inhibition of pain. The neuroendocrine system interacts with the sympathetic and parasympathetic nervous systems as well as the immune system, and thus plays an important role in other dimensions of health and illness such as sleep regulation, fatigue, and responses to stressful events.

neuropathy   Alterations in the function of nerves that are produced by disease or injury. These alterations in function might produce symptoms, such as increased sensitivity with numbness or tingling, pain and burning, decreased sensation, or muscle weakness.

norepinephrine   A neurotransmitter that is produced in the adrenal gland that activates the autonomic nervous system.

NSAIDs   (Nonsteroidal anti-inflammatory drugs). They are used to decrease local areas of inflammation and reduce pain associated with illnesses. These illnesses include rheumatoid arthritis, osteoarthritis, and lupus, among others. Although fibromyalgia is not an inflammatory disease, NSAIDs are sometimes prescribed for people with this condition because NSAIDs may alter pain transmission in the spinal cord or other parts of the central nervous system. However, the response to NSAIDs tends to vary greatly among people with fibromyalgia.

off label   The use of a medication for the treatment of any medical condition other than those specifically approved of by the U.S. Food and Drug Administration. It has been reliably estimated that the vast majority of prescriptions written in the United States (over 70 percent) are written for off-label usage.

overlapping condition   A secondary illness that accompanies the primary illness affecting an individual. Individuals with fibromyalgia are often affected by one or more overlapping illnesses, such as irritable bowel syndrome, chronic tension-type headaches, restless legs syndrome, or interstitial cystitis.

pathophysiology   The study or knowledge of illness or disease as it relates to abnormal physiological (body system) processes. To understand the pathophysiology of a condition is to understand the biological abnormalities that produce its symptoms and the signs associated with it.

polysymptomatic   Characterized by multiple symptoms that frequently involve more than one body system. Fibromyalgia is considered a polysymptomatic disorder because, although the defining characteristic of the disorder is pain, patients are commonly affected by a variety of other symptoms, including fatigue, sleep disturbances, stiffness, cognitive difficulties, and changes in bowel and bladder function (among others).

Raynaud's phenomenon   When blood is restricted from reaching the fingers and toes in response to the cold. The skin turns pale and begins to tingle, becomes numb, and turns painful.

serotonin   A neurotransmitter that modulates mood, emotion, and appetite, aids sleep, and reduces pain.

sleep disorder   A variety of disorders that are associated with changes in sleep habits (for example, difficulty in falling asleep, frequent awakenings from sleep, or reduced quality of sleep or sleep time). These disorders include narcolepsy, insomnia, sleep apnea, restless legs syndrome, and so on. People with fibromyalgia can be affected by any of the dozens of sleep disorders; however, the primary symptom common in fibromyalgia is nonrestorative sleep, or the absence of feeling refreshed upon waking in the morning.

symptom   A perceptible change in a physical or emotional function (for example, pain, shortness of breath, or mood) that reflects an alteration in physiology or health status.

syndrome   A constellation of related symptoms and laboratory test findings.

tender points   Areas of muscle or other soft tissues that are extremely sensitive to pressure stimulation. The American College of Rheumatology criteria for fibromyalgia includes a test in which approximately 4 kilograms of pressure is applied to nine pairs (left side/right side) of tender points. Most healthy individuals experience pain in only a small number of tender points in response to this test. However, one criterion for fibromyalgia is the experience of pain in 11 or more tender points in characteristic locations on the body.

thalamus   A mass of nerve cells located deep in the brain which receives incoming sensory impulses from nerves in the spinal cord. It evokes both physical and emotional reactions.

tissue   A collection of similar cells that act together to perform a specific function of the body.

trigger points   Small areas of muscle that are similar to tender points in that the application of mild pressure produces pain. However, trigger points are characterized by tight bundles of fibers that may refer pain to distant body sites and inhibit contraction or relaxation of the muscle.

unproven remedies   Any treatment that has not been proven safe and effective through repeated scientific studies.

wax and wane   Refers to symptoms that come and go without definitive cause.

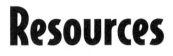

Appendix B

Resources

The following organizations, websites, books, and magazines are exceptionally useful tools that will help you become even more educated about fibromyalgia and overlapping conditions.

National Fibromyalgia Association
www.FMaware.org
714-921-0150

A nonprofit fibromyalgia patient advocacy organization offering a variety of resources aimed at improving the quality of life for people with FM. Includes *Fibromyalgia AWARE* magazine, online newsletters, books, videos, support group contacts, scientific research information, and advocacy concerns.

U.S. Federal Government
www.DisabilityInfo.gov
1-800-333-4636

The federal government's one-stop website for disability-related information, including state and local resources map.

U.S. Social Security Administration
www.ssa.gov
1-800-772-1213

The federal government agency that administers matters related to disability benefits, Supplement Security Income, and Social Security Disability Insurance eligibility.

U.S. Department of Justice
www.ada.gov
1-800-514-0301

The Civil Rights Division Disability Rights Section, which is part of the U.S. Department of Justice, is responsible for enforcing the Americans with Disabilities Act (ADA) and offers information and technical assistance on the ADA.

Patient Advocate Foundation
www.PatientAdvocate.org
1-800-532-5274

The national nonprofit organization helping safeguard patients through effective mediation to assure access to care, maintenance of employment, and preservation of financial stability relative to their diagnosis of life-threatening or debilitating diseases.

National Association of Insurance Commissioners
www.naic.org/state_web_map.htm
1-866-470-NAIC

Offers contact information for each state insurance department. Website users can simply click on their state via a U.S. map to be connected.

U.S. Department of Labor Occupational Safety & Health Administration
www.osha.gov
1-800-321-6742

Helps to ensure employee safety and health in the United States by working with employers and employees to create better working environments.

Organizations

American Academy of Medical Acupuncture
www.medicalacupuncture.org

American Academy of Pain Management
www.aapainmanage.org

American Academy of Pain Medicine
www.painmed.org

American Academy of Physical Medicine and Rehabilitation
www.aapmr.org

American Chiropractic Association
www.amerchiro.org

American Chronic Pain Association
www.theacpa.org

American College of Rheumatology
www.rheumatology.org

American Holistic Medical Association
www.holisticmedicine.org

American Lyme Disease Foundation
www.aldf.com

American Massage Therapy Association
www.amtamassage.org

American Music Therapy Association
www.musictherapy.org

American Occupational Therapy Association
www.aota.org

American Osteopathic Association
www.osteopathic.org

American Pain Society
www.ampainsoc.org

American Physical Therapy Association
www.apta.org

Anxiety Disorders Association of America
www.adaa.org

Association for Applied Psychophysiology and Biofeedback
www.aapb.org

Bureau of Primary Health Care
ask.hrsa.gov/pc

CFIDS Association
www.cfids.org

Depression and Related Affective Disorders Association
www.drada.org

Feldenkrais Guild of North America
www.feldenkrais.com

Fibromyalgia Association UK
www.fibromyalgia-associationuk.org

For Grace-RSD
www.forgrace.org

Hellerwork International
www.hellerwork.com

International Foundation for Functional Gastrointestinal Disorders
www.iffgd.org

International Myopain Society
www.myopain.org

Legal Services Corporation
www.lsc.gov

Lupus Foundation of America
www.lupus.org

Lupus Research Institute
www.lupusresearchinstitute.org

National Association of Cognitive-Behavioral Therapists
www.nacbt.org

National Family Caregivers Association (NFCA)
www.nfcacares.org

National Fibromyalgia Association (NFA)
www.Fmaware.org

National Fibromyalgia Research Association (NFRA)
www.nfra.net

National Headache Foundation
www.headaches.org

National Institute of Arthritis and Musculoskeletal and Skin Disease
www.niams.nih.gov

National Organization of Social Security Claimants' Representatives
www.nosscr.org

National Sleep Foundation
www.sleepfoundation.org

National Women's Health Resource Center
www.healthywomen.org

Oregon Fibromyalgia Foundation
www.myalgia.com

Partnership for Prescription Assistance
www.pparx.org

Patient Advocate Foundation
www.patientadvocate.org

Reflexology Association of America
www.reflexology-usa.org

Restless Legs Syndrome Foundation
www.rls.org

RxHope
www.rxhope.com

Sjögren's Syndrome Foundation
www.sjogrens.org

Temporomandibular Joint Association
www.tmj.org

Together RX Access
www.togetherrxaccess.com

Worldwide Aquatic Bodywork Association
www.waba.edu

Yoga Alliance
www.yogaalliance.org

Informational Websites

Co-Cure
www.co-cure.org

Disability—Scott Davis, Esq.
www.scottdavispc.com/articles.htm

Healing Well-IBS
www.healingwell.com/ibs/

ImmuneSupport.com
www.immunesupport.com/library/showarticle.cfm/ID/3724/e/1/T/CFIDSFM

Medline Plus
www.nlm.nih.gov/medlineplus/fibromyalgia.html

Social Security Online
www.ssa.gov/disability

University of Maryland
www.umm.edu/patiented/articles/what_fibromyalgia_its_symptoms_000076_1.htm

Web MD
www.webmd.com/fibromyalgia/default.htm

Books

Backstrom, Gayle, with Dr. Bernard Rubin. *When Muscle Pain Won't Go Away: The Relief Handbook for Fibromyalgia and Chronic Muscle Pain, Third Edition.* Dallas: Taylor Publishing Company, 1998.

Balch, James F., and Phyllis A Balch. *Prescription for Nutritional Healing: A Practical A–Z Reference to Drug-Free Remedies Using Vitamins, Minerals, Herbs & Food Supplements.* New York: Avery Publishing Group, 2003.

Farhi, Donna. *Breathing Book.* New York: Henry Holt and Company, Inc., 1996.

Fennell, Patricia A., MSW, CSW-R. *Chronic Illness Workbook: Strategies and Solutions for Taking Back Your Life.* Oakland, CA: New Harbinger Publications, Inc., 2001.

Fransen, Jenny, R.N., and I. Jon Russell, M.D., Ph.D. *Fibromyalgia Help Book.* St. Paul, MN: Smith House Press, 1996.

Langenfeld, Carol, and Douglas Langenfeld. *Hope and Encouragement for People with Chronic Illness.* Tucson, AZ: Patient Press, 2001.

Lasater, Judith, Ph.D., P.T. *Relax & Renew.* Berkeley, CA: Rodmell Press, 1995.

Pellegrino, Mark, M.D. *Fibromyalgia Supporter.* Columbus, OH: Anadem Publishing, Inc., 1997.

———. *Fibromyalgia Survivor.* Columbus, OH: Anadem Publishing, Inc., 1995.

———. *From Whiplash to Fibromyalgia.* Columbus, OH: Anadem Publishing, Inc., 2003.

———. *Understanding Post-Traumatic Fibromyalgia.* Columbus, OH: Anadem Publishing, Inc., 1996.

Piburn, Gregg. *Beyond Chaos, One Man's Journey Alongside His Chronically Ill Wife.* Peachtree, GA: Arthritis Foundation, 1999.

Russell, I. Jon, M.D., Ph.D. *Journal of Musculoskeletal Pain.* Binghamton, New York: The Haworth Medical Press, 2003.

Simmons, Kenna. *Natural Treatments for Fibromyalgia.* Peachtree, GA: Arthritis Foundation, 2003.

Teitelbaum, Jacob. *From Fatigued to Fantastic.* New York: Avery, 2001.

Wallace, Daniel J., M.D., and Janice Brock Wallace. *All About Fibromyalgia: A Guide for Patients and Their Families.* New York: Oxford University Press, 2003.

———. *Making Sense of Fibromyalgia: A Guide for Patients and Their Families.* New York: Oxford University Press, 1999.

Magazines

Digestive Health & Nutrition
www.dhn-online.org

Fibromyalgia AWARE
fmaware.org/magazine.html

Journal of Woman's Health
www.liebertpub.com/jwh/default1.asp

Massage Magazine
www.massagemag.com

Yoga Journal
www.yogajournal.com

Medical Journals

Journal of Musculoskeletal Medicine. Greenwich, CT: Cliggott Publishing Co.

Journal of Musculoskeletal Pain. Quarterly publication. Binghamton, NY: Haworth Medical Press.

Journal of the Chronic Fatigue Syndrome. Quarterly publication. Binghamton, NY: Haworth Medical Press.

Conferences

American Academy of Pain Management
www.aapainmanage.org/conference/Conference.php

American College of Rheumatology
www.rheumatology.org/meetings/index.asp?aud=mem

American Pain Society
www.ampainsoc.org/meeting/

National Fibromyalgia Association
fmaware.org/events.htm

Videos

Exercise, Dr. Sharon Clark
www.myalgia.com

For more information on the following videos, call 714-921-0150:

- ◆ *CME: Chronic Pain Management*, NFA
- ◆ *CME: Fibromyalgia*, NFA
- ◆ *A Multidiscipline Approach to Treating Fibromyalgia*, NFA
- ◆ *Opioid Debate*, NFA
- ◆ *Physiological Aspects of Fibromyalgia*, NFA

Appendix C

Forms

This appendix helps you create notes and chart what you experience while developing your self-management program. The ability to track specific activities, people, and thoughts will create a valuable resource for your program. You can also make copies of the following pages and share them with your health-care professional(s), family, and friends. Remember that you can always create your own journal and go into more depth on certain subjects than the space here allows you.

Start with your basic medical information by filling out the information in the Emergency Medical Information form.

Your Emergency Medical Information

Today's date: _____

Name: _____

Address: _____

(Home phone) _____ (Work phone) _____

(Mobile phone) _____

E-mail address: _____

Emergency Contacts

	Name	Phone
Closest relative/ friend:	_____	_____ _____
Second relative/ friend:	_____	_____ _____
Third relative/ friend:	_____	_____ _____
Primary care physician:	_____	_____ _____
Insurance provider:	_____	_____

Medical Information at a Glance

Birth date: _____ Blood type: _____

Height: _____ Weight: _____

Drug allergies: _____

_____

Current Medications

Name	Dose	Frequency
_____	_____	_____
_____	_____	_____
_____	_____	_____
_____	_____	_____
_____	_____	_____

Current medical conditions: _____

_____

_____

_____

Do you have a living will or health-care proxy?　❏ Yes　❏ No

If yes, where is it located? _____

Do you have a Medical Power of Attorney filed?　❏ Yes　❏ No

If yes, where is it located? Agent: _____

Phone: _____

Organ donor?　❏ Yes　❏ No　Donor card ID number: _____

Creating Your Health-Care Team

To keep track of the people who play an important role in your health care, complete the following chart and update it whenever necessary.

My Health-Care Team

Name	Specialty	Address	Phone Number	Web Address E-mail
_____	Medical professionals	_____	_____	_____
_____		_____	_____	_____
_____	Health-care specialists	_____	_____	_____
_____		_____	_____	_____
_____	Pharmacist	_____	_____	_____
_____	Family and friends	_____	_____	_____
_____		_____	_____	_____
_____	Support group members	_____	_____	_____
_____		_____	_____	_____
National Fibromyalgia Association	FM Patient Support and Education/ Fibromyalgia	2121 S. Towne Centre Place, Suite 300, Anaheim, CA 92606	714-921-0150	www.Fmaware.org
AWARE Magazine				www.fmaware.org/site/ PageServer?pagename= resources_ awareMagazine

Medical Records

For future reference, keep a list of each health-care professional you see, hospital stay, laboratory test and/or other medical procedures you take part in. Remember to include all health-care professionals (medical, such as family physician and specialists; alternative, such as acupuncture, massage, and nutritionists; holistic; dental; vision; physical therapists; and so on) and medical tests and procedures (x-rays, MRIs, blood tests, biopsies, and so on).

Date	Health-Care Professional	Specialty	Reason for Appt.	Contact Information
————	————————	————————	—————	————————————
————	————————	————————	—————	————————————
————	————————	————————	—————	————————————
————	————————	————————	—————	————————————
————	————————	————————	—————	————————————
————	————————	————————	—————	————————————

Date	Lab Test Performed	Ordered By	Contact Information
————	————————————	—————	———————————
————	————————————	—————	———————————
————	————————————	—————	———————————
————	————————————	—————	———————————
————	————————————	—————	———————————
————	————————————	—————	———————————
————	————————————	—————	———————————

Date	Medical Procedure/Test	Ordered By	Contact Information
————	————————————	—————	———————————
————	————————————	—————	———————————
————	————————————	—————	———————————
————	————————————	—————	———————————
————	————————————	—————	———————————

Date	Medical Procedure/Test	Ordered By	Contact Information
____	_____	_____	_____
____	_____	_____	_____
____	_____	_____	_____
____	_____	_____	_____
____	_____	_____	_____
____	_____	_____	_____

Date	Type of Injection	Ordered By	Contact Information
____	_____	_____	_____
____	_____	_____	_____
____	_____	_____	_____
____	_____	_____	_____
____	_____	_____	_____

Date	Hospital Stay	Ordered By	Contact Information
____	_____	_____	_____
____	_____	_____	_____
____	_____	_____	_____
____	_____	_____	_____
____	_____	_____	_____

Evaluating Your Family's Communication

In Chapter 5, you identified what communication needs people experience, so you can now identify what needs are or are not being met in your family. Family members should rank each of the following statements on a scale of 1 to 5 (1 being not at all, 2 being rarely, 3 being occasionally, 4 being often, and 5 being all the time). After everyone has contributed to the chart, sit down as a family and address the issues that are positively and negatively affecting each family member.

Family Communication Analysis Chart

Family Members (Including Yourself)

Others in my family listen to me.	1	2	3	4	5
I have at least one attentive listener.	1	2	3	4	5
The members of my family respect what I am telling them.	1	2	3	4	5
I receive verbal emotional support.	1	2	3	4	5
I receive appropriate touch.	1	2	3	4	5
I am able to tell others how their actions affect me without blaming or causing hurt.	1	2	3	4	5
I have a safe place to express my thoughts, feelings, dreams, and aspirations.	1	2	3	4	5
I experience communication that builds self-esteem and creates confidence to take on challenges.	1	2	3	4	5
Others act on my concerns.	1	2	3	4	5
Others invite me into a conversation by asking me a question.	1	2	3	4	5
I am reassured that I am loved.	1	2	3	4	5

Family Members (Including Yourself)

I have the opportunity to talk to others who know what I am going through.	1	2	3	4	5
I am not afraid to express my true feelings.	1	2	3	4	5
I listen to members of my family.	1	2	3	4	5
Others in my family encourage me to express myself.	1	2	3	4	5
I never say things that aren't true just to protect someone else's feelings.	1	2	3	4	5
If I feel the need to discuss a specific topic with my family, I feel comfortable addressing the subject with them.	1	2	3	4	5
I experience communication that involves laughing and having fun.	1	2	3	4	5
I feel I am accepted for the person I am.	1	2	3	4	5

Medications Diary

Following are three diaries to track medications, complementary or alternative therapies, and treatments for overlapping conditions that you have tried and whether you found them to be helpful.

Medication: _____ Dosage: _____

Health-care professional: _____

Treatment for what symptom: _____ Start date: _____ End date: _____

Positive benefits: _____

_____

_____

Negative benefits: _____

_____

_____

Medication: _____ Dosage: _____

Health-care professional: _____

Treatment for what symptom: _____ Start date: _____ End date: _____

Positive benefits: _____

_____

_____

Negative benefits: _____

_____

_____

Medication: _____ Dosage: _____

Health-care professional: _____

Treatment for what symptom: _____ Start date: _____ End date: _____

Positive benefits: _____

_____

_____

Negative benefits: _____

_____

_____

Medication: _____   Dosage: _____

Health-care professional: _____

Treatment for what symptom: _____   Start date: _____   End date: _____

Positive benefits: _____

_____

_____

Negative benefits: _____

_____

_____

Complementary and Alternative Therapies Diary

Therapy: _____   Health-care professional: _____

Specific treatment info: _____

Treatment for what symptom: _____   Start date: _____   End date: _____

Positive benefits: _____

_____

_____

Negative benefits: _____

_____

_____

Therapy: _____   Health-care professional: _____

Specific treatment info: _____

Treatment for what symptom: _____   Start date: _____   End date: _____

Positive benefits: _____

_____

_____

Negative benefits: _____

_____

_____

Therapy: _____ Health-care professional: _____

Specific treatment info: _____

Treatment for what symptom: _____ Start date: _____ End date: _____

Positive benefits: _____

_____

_____

Negative benefits: _____

_____

_____

Therapy: _____ Health-care professional: _____

Specific treatment info: _____

Treatment for what symptom: _____ Start date: _____ End date: _____

Positive benefits: _____

_____

_____

Negative benefits: _____

_____

_____

Overlapping Conditions Treatment Diary

Condition: _____ Health-care professional: _____

Medication: _____ Dosage: _____

Treatment for what symptom: _____ Start date: _____ End date: _____

Positive benefits: _____

_____

_____

Negative benefits: _____

_____

_____

Condition: _____   Health-care professional: _____

Medication: _____   Dosage: _____

Treatment for what symptom: _____   Start date: _____   End date: _____

Positive benefits: _____

_____

_____

Negative benefits: _____

_____

_____

Condition: _____   Health-care professional: _____

Medication: _____   Dosage: _____

Treatment for what symptom: _____   Start date: _____   End date: _____

Positive benefits: _____

_____

_____

Negative benefits: _____

_____

_____

Condition: _____   Health-care professional: _____

Medication: _____   Dosage: _____

Treatment for what symptom: _____   Start date: _____   End date: _____

Positive benefits: _____

_____

_____

Negative benefits: _____

_____

_____

Condition: _____   Health-care professional: _____

Medication: _____   Dosage: _____

Treatment for what symptom: _____   Start date: _____   End date: _____

Positive benefits: _____

_____

_____

Negative benefits: _____

_____

_____

Personal Plan for Lifestyle Changes

In this chart, you can select and then list certain activities or practices that you feel you should change to improve your lifestyle.

Example: Eliminate activities that are not healthy.

1. Reduce my coffee intake to one cup with breakfast.
   Start date: Immediately

2. Try to do stretching exercises daily.
   Start date: Immediately

3. Do not lift anything heavy that increases my pain.
   Start date: Immediately

Improve my sleep habits.

1. _____
   Start date: _____

2. _____
   Start date: _____

3. _____
   Start date: _____

4. _____
   Start date: _____

5. _____

Start date: _____

6. _____

Start date: _____

Exercise as often as possible.

1. _____

Start date: _____

2. _____

Start date: _____

3. _____

Start date: _____

4. _____

Start date: _____

5. _____

Start date: _____

6. _____

Start date: _____

Change my diet.

1. _____

Start date: _____

2. _____

Start date: _____

3. _____

Start date: _____

4. _____

Start date: _____

5. _____

Start date: _____

6. _____

Start date: _____

Learn how to relax and enjoy quiet and self-reflection time.

1. _____
   Start date: _____

2. _____
   Start date: _____

3. _____
   Start date: _____

4. _____
   Start date: _____

5. _____
   Start date: _____

6. _____
   Start date: _____

Conserve personal energy.

1. _____
   Start date: _____

2. _____
   Start date: _____

3. _____
   Start date: _____

4. _____
   Start date: _____

5. _____
   Start date: _____

6. _____
   Start date: _____

7. _____
   Start date: _____

8. _____
   Start date: _____

Eliminate activities or foods that are unhealthy (for example, caffeine and alcohol).

1. _____
   Start date: _____

2. _____
   Start date: _____

3. _____
   Start date: _____

4. _____
   Start date: _____

5. _____
   Start date: _____

6. _____
   Start date: _____

Shift my focus and establish new priorities.

1. _____
   Start date: _____

2. _____
   Start date: _____

3. _____
   Start date: _____

4. _____
   Start date: _____

5. _____
   Start date: _____

6. _____
   Start date: _____

7. _____
   Start date: _____

8. _____
   Start date: _____

Adjust the importance I place on things that do not matter.

1. _____

   Start date: _____

2. _____

   Start date: _____

3. _____

   Start date: _____

4. _____

   Start date: _____

5. _____

   Start date: _____

6. _____

   Start date: _____

7. _____

   Start date: _____

8. _____

   Start date: _____

Make sense out of my life's new purpose.

1. _____

   Start date: _____

2. _____

   Start date: _____

3. _____

   Start date: _____

4. _____

   Start date: _____

5. _____

   Start date: _____

6. _____

   Start date: _____

Take part in activities that focus on my own emotional well-being.

1. _____

   Start date: _____

2. _____

   Start date: _____

3. _____

   Start date: _____

4. _____

   Start date: _____

5. _____

   Start date: _____

6. _____

   Start date: _____

Health Care Provider Patient Appointment Preparation Form

Here is a quick and easy form for you to prepare before your next doctor's appointment. This information will provide an accurate and organized accounting of your symptoms and concerns. Be prepared, save time, and ensure good communication with your health-care provider!

Name: _____   Date: _____

Medications you are allergic to or cannot tolerate: _____

_____

Current Medications (name, amount, how often taken):

_____

_____

_____

Problems with Current Medications (side effects, discontinuation, changes in amounts or when taken): _____

_____

_____

Current Supplements/Herbs (name, amount, how often taken, effectiveness):

_____

_____

_____

Activity Level (past week): ❏ High ❏ Medium ❏ Low ❏ None

Quality of Sleep (the amount of sleep you get, quality, number of times you wake up in the night, how long you stay awake, other issues related to sleep):

_____

_____

Pain Level (past week):

Scale of 1–10 (10 being worst possible) _____ Is this an improvement? ❏ Yes ❏ No

Duration, type, and lifestyle changes due to pain: _____

_____

Physical and Emotional Symptoms: (if you need more room, list on a separate sheet of paper): _____

_____

_____

_____

_____

_____

_____

_____

_____

Symptom (date of onset, frequency level of adversity, how much is this affecting your life?) _____

_____

_____

Questions and Concerns: (Limit number to 3.)

   1.

   2.

   3.

Information you want your doctor to know:

1.

2.

3.

4.

5.

Note: It can be helpful to have someone attend your appointment with you to take notes and listen to what the doctor says. Always be open and direct with your doctor, and remember the relationship will be most successful if you create a partnership with your doctor.

Index

I

X-Y-Z

...k out these

READ BY MILLIONS!

BEST-SELLERS

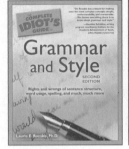

Grammar and Style
SECOND EDITION

Rights and wrongs of sentence structure, word usage, spelling, and much, much more

Laurie E. Rozakis, Ph.D.

978-1-59257-115-4
$16.95

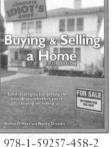

Buying & Selling a Home
FIFTH EDITION

Solid strategies for getting the best deal—whether you're buying or selling

Shelley O'Hara and Nancy D. Lewis

978-1-59257-458-2
$19.95

FULL COLOR!

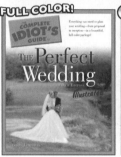

The Perfect Wedding

978-1-59257-566-4
$22.95

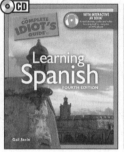

Learning Spanish
FOURTH EDITION

Gail Stein

978-1-59257-485-8
$24.95

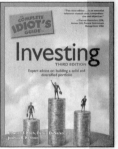

Investing
THIRD EDITION

Expert advice on building a solid and diversified portfolio

Edward T. Koch, Debra DeSalvo, Joshua A. Kennon

978-1-59257-480-3
$19.95

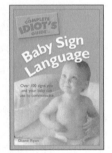

Baby Sign Language

Over 100 signs you and your baby can use to communicate

Diane Ryan

978-1-59257-469-8
$14.95

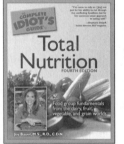

Total Nutrition
FOURTH EDITION

Food group fundamentals from the dairy, fruit, vegetable, and grain worlds

Joy Bauer, M.S., R.D., C.D.N.

978-1-59257-439-1
$18.95

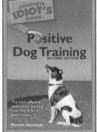

Positive Dog Training
SECOND EDITION

The most effective method for teaching your dog to be a good citizen

Pamela Dennison

978-1-59257-483-4
$14.95

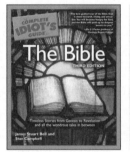

The Bible
THIRD EDITION

Timeless Stories from Genesis to Revelation

James Stuart Bell and Stan Campbell

978-1-59257-389-9
$18.95

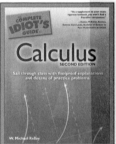

Calculus
SECOND EDITION

Sail through class with foolproof explanations and dozens of practice problems

W. Michael Kelley

978-1-59257-471-1
$18.95

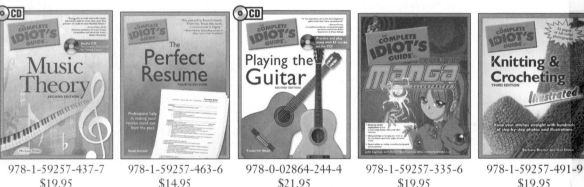

Music Theory
SECOND EDITION

Michael Miller

978-1-59257-437-7
$19.95

The Perfect Resume
FOURTH EDITION

Professional help in making your resume stand out from the pack

Susan Ireland

978-1-59257-463-6
$14.95

Playing the Guitar
SECOND EDITION

Frederick Noad

978-0-02864-244-4
$21.95

MANGA
ILLUSTRATED

John Layman and David Hutchison

978-1-59257-335-6
$19.95

Knitting & Crocheting
THIRD EDITION
Illustrated

Keep your stitches straight with hundreds of step-by-step photos and illustrations

Barbara Breiter and Gail Diven

978-1-59257-491-9
$19.95

More than **450 titles** available at booksellers and online retailers everywhere

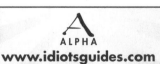

ALPHA

www.idiotsguides.com